Psychics

How to Develop Your Inner Psychic Power

(The Modern Guide to Psychic Self Defence With Crystals for Empaths)

Bernard Bolick

Published By **John Kembrey**

Bernard Bolick

All Rights Reserved

Psychics: How to Develop Your Inner Psychic Power (The Modern Guide to Psychic Self Defence With Crystals for Empaths)

ISBN 978-1-7780570-2-1

No part of this guidebook shall be reproduced in any form without permission in writing from the publisher except in the case of brief quotations embodied in critical articles or reviews.

Legal & Disclaimer

The information contained in this book is not designed to replace or take the place of any form of medicine or professional medical advice. The information in this book has been provided for educational & entertainment purposes only.

The information contained in this book has been compiled from sources deemed reliable, and it is accurate to the best of the Author's knowledge; however, the Author cannot guarantee its accuracy and validity and cannot be held liable for any errors or omissions. Changes are periodically made to this book. You must consult your doctor or get professional medical advice before using any of the suggested remedies, techniques, or information in this book.

Upon using the information contained in this book, you agree to hold harmless the Author from and against any damages, costs, and expenses, including any legal fees potentially resulting from the application of any of the information provided by this guide. This disclaimer applies to any damages or injury caused by the use and application, whether directly or indirectly, of any advice or information presented, whether for breach of contract, tort, negligence, personal injury, criminal intent, or under any other cause of action.

You agree to accept all risks of using the information presented inside this book. You need to consult a professional medical practitioner in order to ensure you are both able and healthy enough to participate in this program.

Table Of Contents

Chapter 1: What Is Psychic Energy? 1

Chapter 2: The Best Psychic Love Spells . 14

Chapter 3: Psychic Surgery At The Etheric Body 32

Chapter 4: The Bridge Between The Psychic And The Veil 40

Chapter 5: Sigils 79

Chapter 6: Historical Psychic Oppression 92

Chapter 7: Astral Projection Guidelines 111

Chapter 8: Are Mediums And Psychics The Identical Element? 129

Chapter 9: Energy First! 134

Chapter 10: Am I Psychic? 145

Chapter 11: Am I A Medium? 171

Chapter 1: What Is Psychic Energy?

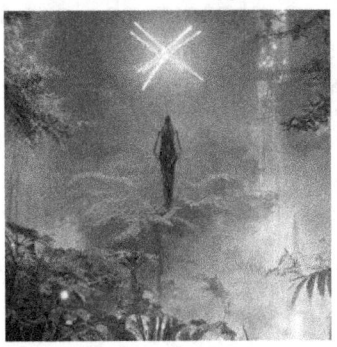

Psychic energy is a subtle power that surrounds and permeates all dwelling beings and items. It is likewise called psi energy, lifestyles pressure electricity, or chi power. This energy is thought to be the underlying strain that connects all things in the universe, together with human beings, animals, flora, or maybe inanimate devices. Psychic energy is said to be chargeable for psychic phenomena along with telepathy, clairvoyance, and precognition.

Notable Psychic Abilities:

Clairvoyance: The capability to appearance subjects beyond the physical realm, which include visions, photographs, or symbols.

Clairaudience: The potential to concentrate topics past the physical realm, alongside facet voices, track, or sounds.

Clairsentience: The functionality to revel in or sense subjects past the physical realm, at the side of feelings, energies, or vibrations.

Telepathy: The capacity to examine or transmit mind and feelings amongst two or more people without the use of physical senses.

Precognition: The potential to recognize future sports activities or situations in advance than they appear.

Psychokinesis: The potential to transport or manipulate devices with the energy of the mind.

Mediumship: The potential to communicate with spirits or entities from the afterlife.

Astral Projection: The capability to split the attention from the physical frame and adventure through special dimensions or planes of existence.

Empathy: The capacity to revel in and understand the feelings of others.

Healing: The functionality to use psychic power to heal physical or emotional ailments in oneself or others.

To enlarge and enhance the ones capabilities, one should exercise and teach the mind via meditation, visualization, and psychic spells. With time and determination, it's miles possible to free up the whole ability of psychic electricity and harness its energy to reap effective consequences in a unmarried's lifestyles.

How to tap into your energy

Relax and clean your mind: To access your psychic power, it is important to easy your thoughts of any distracting thoughts and loosen up your frame. You can try this via deep breathing, meditation, or visualization.

Focus for your instinct: Your intuition is your inner guidance system that allow you to faucet into your psychic energy. Focus to your intestine feelings and pay attention on your inner voice. Trust your instinct and use it as a tool to get right of get entry to to your psychic strength.

Practice mindfulness: Mindfulness is the exercising of being gift inside the 2d and absolutely aware about your thoughts, emotions, and sensations. This will let you boom a deeper reference to your psychic electricity and enhance your psychic competencies.

Use psychic tools: There are many system you can use to help you tap into your psychic strength, which include crystals, tarot playing cards, pendulums, or runes. Choose the tool that resonates with you and use it to help you get proper of get right of entry to in your psychic energy.

Practice visualization: Visualization is a powerful tool for gaining access to your psychic energy. Imagine a beam of mild or energy flowing through your frame, beginning at your toes and shifting up through the pinnacle of your head. Visualize this energy growing and filling your air of mystery.

Connect with nature: Spending time in nature will assist you to hook up with your psychic electricity. Take a walk inside the woods, take a seat via a river or ocean, or absolutely spend time to your lawn. Allow yourself to emerge as actually immersed within the herbal global and revel in the electricity that surrounds you.

Remember that tapping into your psychic energy requires workout and staying power. It's critical to increase a everyday habitual of meditation, visualization, and different practices that will help you get proper of entry in your psychic capabilities. With dedication and staying energy, you can unencumber the complete capability of your psychic strength and use it to acquire splendid consequences in your life.

How to ground into the earth to raise vibration

Grounding is a effective technique that lets in you hook up with the Earth's power and lift your vibration. Here are a few steps you could study to floor into the Earth:

Find a quiet and peaceful vicinity: Look for a quiet and non violent location in which you may take a seat down or stand surely with out being disturbed.

Take deep breaths: Take a few deep breaths and recognition in your breath. Feel the air moving internal and from your frame and permit move of any anxiety or stress.

Visualize roots: Visualize roots growing from the soles of your ft or the bottom of your spine, extending deep into the Earth. Imagine these roots reaching right all the way down to the Earth's middle, connecting you to the electricity of the planet.

Use affirmations: Use affirmations to help you connect to the Earth's power. Repeat terms which incorporates "I am grounded and related to the Earth's electricity" or "I am one with the Earth's vibrations."

Connect with nature: Spend time in nature that will help you connect with the Earth's power. Take a walk inside the woods, sit through a river or ocean, or definitely spend time to your garden. Allow your self to emerge as honestly immersed inside the herbal global and feel the energy that surrounds you.

Practice gratitude: Expressing gratitude for the Earth's objects allow you to hook up with its power. Take a second to thank the Earth for its splendor and abundance, and sense a enjoy of appreciation and love for the planet.

Remember that grounding is a exercising that calls for ordinary interest and focus. By grounding into the Earth, you can enhance your vibration and experience more related to the herbal international. This will let you gain extra clarity, peace, and concord for your life.

The Auramagnet Theory (TAT)

The Auramagnet Theory is my personal:

A precept that shows that paying attention to geomagnetic solar storms may also have a direct effect at the frame and psychic powers. This concept is primarily based on the idea that these storms can reason adjustments within the Earth's magnetic discipline, which in flip will have an impact on the human body and its energy vicinity or air of mystery.

According to this principle, the Earth's magnetic field and the human air of mystery are interconnected. The human charisma is a diffused power concern that surrounds the body and is made of various layers or frequencies of power. It is belief that the air of mystery is stricken by the Earth's magnetic concern, which could impact the steadiness and drift of strength inside the body.

Geomagnetic sun storms are because of eruptions at the floor of the sun that release big portions of electricity and particles into location. When those debris interact with the Earth's magnetic area, they will be able to purpose fluctuations and disturbances in the task. These disturbances can be measured via way of devices along with magnetometers and are called geomagnetic storms.

The Auramagnet Theory shows that when those storms rise up, they could have an immediate effect on the human body and its power area. Some people don't forget that those storms can enhance psychic capabilities, collectively with clairvoyance, telepathy, and intuition. It is belief that the accelerated power and frequency of the storms can stimulate the electricity facilities of the frame, which includes the chakras, and help to growth and beautify psychic powers.

There is some scientific evidence to assist the idea that geomagnetic storms might also have an impact at the body and thoughts. Studies have examined that those storms can motive changes in mind hobby, temper, and conduct. Some human beings record feeling extra energized and alert during those storms, at the same time as others also can experience headaches, dizziness, or distinct bodily signs and symptoms and symptoms and symptoms and symptoms.

In quit, TAT suggests that taking note of geomagnetic sun storms can have a right away impact at the body and psychic powers. While there's despite the fact that a bargain to be understood approximately the relationship among the Earth's magnetic scenario and the human air of secrecy, it's far smooth that those forces are in detail associated and can have a sizable effect on our fitness and nicely-being.

The Best Psychic Defense Spells

Psychic protection spells can be a effective tool for protective your self in competition to negative power, psychic assaults, and other styles of harm. There are many excellent styles of psychic protection spells, each with its own unique houses and strategies of use. In this financial ruin, we're capable of find out some of the excellent psychic safety spells and how to use them efficiently.

Protection Spell: The Protection Spell is one of the maximum number one and powerful psychic protection spells. To perform this spell, surely visualize a shield of white moderate surrounding you and defensive you from harm. You can also use a physical item, which includes a piece of jewellery or a crystal, to characteristic a talisman of safety.

Salt Circle Spell: The Salt Circle Spell is a few different clean but effective psychic protection spell. To carry out this spell, sprinkle a circle of salt around your self or your own home, visualizing the salt forming a protective barrier in opposition to terrible power and psychic attacks.

Mirror Spell: The Mirror Spell is a defensive spell that suggests awful electricity lower back to its source. To carry out this spell, visualize a reflect inside the front of you and interest on reflecting any awful electricity or psychic attacks again to their deliver.

Binding Spell: The Binding Spell is a protective spell that binds poor power or entities and stops them from harming you. To carry out this spell, visualize a twine or ribbon binding the horrible power or entity, and repeat a binding incantation which consist of "I bind you, I banish you, I ship you away."

Banishing Spell: The Banishing Spell is a effective shielding spell that eliminates terrible electricity or entities from your surroundings. To perform this spell, visualize the horrific electricity or entity leaving your vicinity, and repeat a banishing incantation which incorporates "Be lengthy lengthy long past, be banished, depart this location."

Cleansing Spell: The Cleansing Spell is a protective spell that eliminates awful power from your charisma or environment. To carry out this spell, visualize a white slight cleansing and purifying your air of mystery or area, and repeat a cleaning incantation which encompass "I cleanse and purify this place, getting rid of all negativity."

Warding Spell: The Warding Spell is a protective spell that creates a barrier of electricity round your area or air of thriller, stopping bad power or entities from coming into. To perform this spell, visualize a defend or barrier of electricity spherical your location or air of thriller, and repeat a warding incantation which encompass "I ward this area, protecting it from all damage."

When performing any psychic safety spell, it's miles essential to focus your goal and power for your desired final results. You also can use bodily items, which embody crystals or candles, to enhance the power of your spells. Remember that psychic protection spells are a effective device for protecting your self, but they will be now not an alternative preference to searching out expert assist or addressing underlying problems that may be causing poor power on your life.

Chapter 2: The Best Psychic Love Spells

Psychic love spells are spells that use psychic electricity to assist lure, enhance, or deepen romantic love. These spells may be used to decorate present relationships or to attract new love into your existence. However, it's far important to remember that at the equal time as psychic love spells may be a effective device, they need to in no manner be used to govern or control some different character's loose will.

There are many actually one among a type types of psychic love spells, each with its very very very own specific homes and strategies of use. In this economic catastrophe, we're capable of discover a number of the maximum well-known psychic love spells and the way to apply them efficiently.

Attraction Spell: The Attraction Spell is a easy however effective psychic love spell that is designed to help you appeal to a today's love hobby. To carry out this spell, you could need a red or crimson candle and a few rose petals.

Light the candle and sprinkle the rose petals round it. Focus your cause on attracting a contemporary love hobby into your lifestyles, and visualize yourself in a happy, loving relationship. Let the candle burn down really.

Binding Spell: The Binding Spell is a powerful psychic love spell this is used to deepen the emotional connection amongst humans. To perform this spell, you could want a crimson or purple candle and a few hair or a personal object from every you and your accomplice. Light the candle and maintain the devices in your hands, focusing your reason on deepening your emotional connection. Visualize a white slight surrounding both you and your accomplice, connecting you every on a deep emotional degree. Let the candle burn down absolutely.

Reconciliation Spell: The Reconciliation Spell is a psychic love spell this is designed to help mend a damaged courting or reunite with an ex-partner. To perform this spell, you could need a red or pink candle and a photo or private object out of your ex-associate. Light the candle and maintain the image or item to your palms, focusing your intention on reuniting together along with your ex-companion and recovery any past hurts. Visualize a white slight surrounding each you and your ex-partner, recuperation any emotional wounds and bringing you returned collectively. Let the candle burn down definitely.

Passion Spell: The Passion Spell is a psychic love spell that is designed to decorate the physical and emotional ardour amongst people. To perform this spell, you can need a purple candle and some cinnamon oil. Anoint the candle with the cinnamon oil, focusing your purpose on improving the ardour among you and your companion. Light the candle and visualize the flame igniting a spark of ardour internal every you and your companion. Let the candle burn down sincerely.

Commitment Spell: The Commitment Spell is a psychic love spell this is used to encourage a partner to decide to a protracted-time period courting. To perform this spell, you could need a red or purple candle and a few parchment paper. Write your associate's call at the parchment paper and place it underneath the candle. Light the candle and reputation your motive on encouraging your companion to determine to an extended-time period courting. Visualize a white slight surrounding every you and your accomplice, deepening your emotional connection and inspiring determination. Let the candle burn down in fact.

When acting any psychic love spell, it's far crucial to bear in mind that those spells need to be used ethically and responsibly. They should in no way be used to control or manage every different man or woman's unfastened will, and that they've to usually be finished with the very exquisite intentions of love and wonderful energy. Remember to usually searching for recommendation from a professional in case you are experiencing any courting or emotional issues that can be negatively impacting your life.

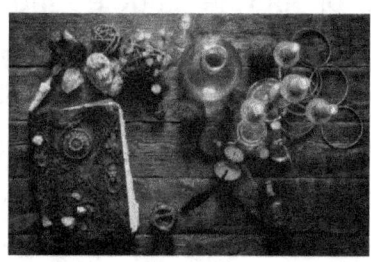

Psychic Success Spells

Psychic achievement spells are spells that use psychic strength to help advantage success in extraordinary elements of lifestyles. These spells may be used to draw abundance, profession success, financial balance, or a few other form of fulfillment. However, it's far critical to keep in mind that whilst psychic fulfillment spells may be a effective tool, they have to in no way be used to damage others or for egocentric abilties.

There are many first rate varieties of psychic achievement spells, every with its very very personal particular houses and techniques of use. In this financial ruin, we are able to explore a number of the maximum famous psychic success spells and a manner to use them efficaciously.

Abundance Spell: The Abundance Spell is a psychic success spell this is designed to attract abundance into your lifestyles. To carry out this spell, you may want a green candle and a few patchouli oil. Anoint the candle with the patchouli oil, focusing your intention on attracting abundance and prosperity into your lifestyles. Light the candle and visualize yourself surrounded via abundance and prosperity. Let the candle burn down simply.

Career Success Spell: The Career Success Spell is a psychic achievement spell this is used to attract profession achievement and development. To perform this spell, you may want a yellow candle and some bergamot oil. Anoint the candle with the bergamot oil, focusing your purpose on undertaking profession fulfillment and development. Light the candle and visualize your self in a successful and fun career. Let the candle burn down honestly.

Financial Stability Spell: The Financial Stability Spell is a psychic fulfillment spell this is designed to attract economic stability and protection. To carry out this spell, you may need a green candle and a few cinnamon oil. Anoint the candle with the cinnamon oil, focusing your goal on attracting economic balance and security. Light the candle and visualize yourself surrounded via financial abundance and safety. Let the candle burn down surely.

Confidence Spell: The Confidence Spell is a psychic achievement spell this is used to decorate self-self guarantee and shallowness. To perform this spell, you can need a yellow candle and some lemon oil. Anoint the candle with the lemon oil, focusing your goal on boosting self-self belief and vanity. Light the candle and visualize your self feeling assured and self-confident in any situation. Let the candle burn down certainly.

Manifestation Spell: The Manifestation Spell is a psychic fulfillment spell that is designed to assist show up your dreams and goals. To carry out this spell, you will want a white candle and some lavender oil. Anoint the candle with the lavender oil, focusing your purpose on manifesting your desires and dreams. Light the candle and visualize your self attaining your desires and dreams. Let the candle burn down surely.

When performing any psychic achievement spell, it's miles vital to endure in thoughts that those spells should be used ethically and responsibly. They must in no manner be used to harm others or for selfish features, and they should commonly be finished with the terrific intentions of positivity and fulfillment. Remember to usually seek advice from a professional in case you are experiencing any problems on your existence that may be negatively impacting your success.

Protect Your Energy Field

Protecting your electricity issue is an essential exercising for retaining your psychic and emotional nicely-being. Your electricity problem, additionally known as your air of thriller, is the subtle strength that surrounds your body and can be inspired with the resource of the power of others or the surroundings around you. Here are a few tactics to defend your electricity region:

Visualize a Protective Bubble: One of the handiest approaches to defend your power task is to visualise a protective bubble around you. This bubble can be fabricated from any fabric or coloration that resonates with you, collectively with white moderate, gold, or pink. Envision the bubble truly surrounding you and recollect it blocking out any awful or harmful electricity.

Use Protective Crystals: Certain crystals, at the facet of black tourmaline, amethyst, or hematite, can assist shield your power discipline. You can deliver the ones crystals with you, put on them as earrings, or area them to your environment to take in any horrible strength.

Create Boundaries: Creating limitations is an crucial part of shielding your power difficulty. You can try this through announcing "no" to people or conditions that drain your electricity, or via the usage of limiting your exposure to terrible environments or humans.

Cleanse Your Energy: Regularly cleansing your electricity can assist get rid of any terrible or stagnant strength out of your energy region. You can try this thru practices along with meditation, yoga, smudging with sage or palo santo, or taking a salt tub.

Use Protective Mantras: Repeating a protecting mantra, which consist of "I am surrounded through superb electricity and safety," can help make stronger your power location and thrust back any terrible energy.

It is crucial to remember that protecting your strength trouble is a private workout, and what works for one man or woman may not artwork for every other. It is important to check with splendid strategies and find out what resonates with you. With everyday exercise, you could deliver a boost to your power location and maintain your psychic and emotional nicely-being.

Written in the Stars

Here are some famous psychics and their extremely good abilties:

Allison Dubois: Dubois is an American psychic medium who is recognized for her ability to speak with the deceased. She has assisted law enforcement businesses in fixing crimes and has written severa books approximately her testimonies.

Edgar Cayce: Cayce, also referred to as the "Sleeping Prophet," become an American psychic who claimed to have the capability to get proper of get entry to to the Akashic Records, a compendium of understanding that includes facts approximately every soul and its adventure thru time. Cayce gave hundreds of psychic readings all through his life, hundreds of which may be however studied and used nowadays.

Theresa Caputo: Caputo is a New York-based totally definitely completely psychic medium who is recognized for her reality TV show "Long Island Medium." She claims on the manner to speak with the vain and has carried out readings for lots celebrities and public figures.

John Edward: Edward is an American psychic medium who's stated for his functionality to speak with the useless. He has written numerous books approximately his opinions and has regarded on severa TV shows.

James Van Praagh: Van Praagh is an American psychic medium who is recognized for his potential to talk with the lifeless. He has written numerous books and has hosted TV suggests and stay events.

Sylvia Browne: Browne changed into an American psychic who claimed to have the capacity to speak with the deceased and to peer into the future. She wrote numerous books and made numerous TV appearances all through her career.

Uri Geller: Geller is an Israeli psychic who's regarded for his potential to bend spoons and perform extraordinary acts of telekinesis. He has also claimed at the way to examine minds and anticipate the destiny.

It is important to word that at the same time as these people are famous for his or her psychic competencies, there can be frequently controversy and skepticism surrounding their claims. It is as lots as all people to decide their private ideals approximately psychic abilities and those who declare to very own them.

Psychic Tools to Consider

Psychic gear are devices or techniques that may be used to beautify psychic abilities or to beneficial useful resource in divination. Here are a few common psychic gadget and their information:

Tarot Cards: Tarot gambling playing playing cards are a deck of gambling playing cards with severa symbolic pix that may be used for divination. Each card has a completely particular due to this and may offer notion into a person's past, gift, and future.

Runes: Runes are a fixed of symbols that have been utilized in historical times for divination. They are frequently inscribed on small stones or quantities of wood and are believed to have unique meanings.

Crystals: Crystals are believed to have restoration and psychic houses. They may be used for meditation, energy work, or to enhance psychic abilities. Each crystal has a totally particular energy and may be used for precise purposes.

Pendulums: Pendulums are small gadgets, frequently made from crystal or metallic, which is probably suspended on a chain or cord. They may be used to answer sure or no questions or to offer steering.

Scrying Mirrors: Scrying mirrors are used for divination and are often made from black obsidian or other reflective materials. They can be used to analyze the destiny or to advantage insight proper right into a situation.

Astrology: Astrology is the take a look at of the moves and positions of celestial our bodies and their effect on human affairs. Astrology may be used for divination or to advantage insight into someone's persona or life direction.

Numerology: Numerology is the examine of numbers and their importance. It may be used for divination or to gain belief into a person's personality or existence route.

Psychometry: Psychometry is the capability to have a look at the electricity of an item or man or woman thru touching it. Psychometry can be used to gain perception into someone's beyond, gift, or destiny.

Aura Readings: Aura readings are a way used to take a look at a person's air of thriller, that is the diffused power that surrounds their body. An air of secrecy analyzing can provide notion into someone's emotional, mental, and bodily nicely-being.

It is crucial to notice that at the same time as those system can be useful for enhancing psychic competencies or gaining perception, they ought to no longer be relied upon completely for preference making or existence selections. It is crucial to use the ones system at the facet of your private intuition and not unusual feel.

Trauma Related Psychic Stress- Telekinesis, Telepathy and Other Abilities

Trauma may additionally need to have a massive effect on someone's psychic abilities, on the facet of telekinesis, telepathy, and particular abilties. Here are some tactics that trauma will have an effect on psychic capabilities:

Telekinesis: Trauma can block the go along with the glide of electricity within the body, that might inhibit the ability to perform telekinetic acts. Additionally, trauma can result in emotions of helplessness or lack of manage, that could make it tough to popularity and deliver interest to telekinetic responsibilities.

Telepathy: Trauma can motive emotional distress and make it tough to trust others, that could effect the capacity to acquire and interpret telepathic messages. Additionally, trauma can cause feelings of isolation and detachment, which could make it hard to connect to others on a psychic stage.

Other Abilities: Trauma can also have an effect on remarkable psychic abilties, which include clairvoyance, clairaudience, and precognition. Trauma can purpose heightened anxiety, strain, and fear, that may make it tough to access the ones abilties. Additionally, trauma can impact a person's sense of self, which can have an impact on their potential to believe their private instinct and psychic insights.

It is crucial for humans who've professional trauma to are attempting to find expert help at the manner to deal with the underlying emotional and intellectual problems that may be impacting their psychic abilties. Therapy, meditation, and energy recuperation practices can all be useful in lowering stress and anxiety, and in restoring balance to the body's electricity systems. Additionally, human beings can work on strengthening their psychic skills with the aid of operating towards grounding and visualization strategies, and through jogging with depended on mentors or publications within the psychic network.

Chapter 3: Psychic Surgery At The Etheric Body

Psychic surgery is a shape of energy healing that consists of the elimination of terrible energy or entities from someone's strength discipline. When completed at the etheric frame, it's miles known as etheric psychic surgical remedy.

The etheric body is the strength body that surrounds the physical frame and is thought to be accountable for retaining physical health and well-being. When the etheric frame is damaged or blocked, it can rise up as physical or emotional troubles within the bodily body.

Etheric psychic surgical treatment consists of a psychic healer the usage of their fingers or other device to govern the power challenge across the body. They may additionally additionally furthermore use visualization, goal, or distinctive strength healing strategies to perceive and eliminate horrible power or entities from the etheric frame. This can assist to repair stability to the power region and sell bodily and emotional healing.

Some of the benefits of etheric psychic surgical treatment encompass:

Relief from bodily pain and pain

Reduction of emotional pressure and tension

Improved energy ranges and strength

Increased clarity and reputation

Accelerated restoration from infection or damage

It is crucial to word that whilst etheric psychic surgical procedure can be beneficial in promoting recovery and well-being, it need to not be relied upon as an alternative for clinical or mental treatment. Individuals want to commonly are attempting to find the recommendation of a licensed healthcare expert for any bodily or intellectual health issues.

Additionally, it's far essential to paintings with a relied on and expert psychic healer at the same time as receiving etheric psychic surgical remedy. It is crucial to research and pick out out a practitioner who has a wonderful reputation and who you revel in comfortable going for walks with.

Spiritual Red Flags, Invading Entities and Possession

Please be responsible even as coping with your items to help others.

When having to address a possession- list the signs and symptoms of ownership and make a clean rationalization of the consequences of poor psychic safety

Dealing with possession may be a severe and hard situation. Here are a few signs and symptoms and signs of ownership and the results of bad psychic protection:

Signs of Possession:

Changes in conduct or character

Loss of memory or awareness

Unexplained physical injuries or markings

Hearing voices or seeing apparitions

Sudden onset of despair or tension

Uncontrollable mood swings or emotional outbursts

Extreme fatigue or insomnia

Suicidal thoughts or behaviors

Changes in consuming or slumbering conduct

Sensitivity to moderate or sound

Consequences of Poor Psychic Defense:

Physical harm to the person or others

Damage to personal relationships

Financial or crook effects

Permanent harm to the character's psychic or religious nicely-being

Permanent lack of control over one's very personal body and movements

Increased threat of bad psychic testimonies and encounters

Increased threat of intellectual and emotional disorders

Decreased remarkable of life and standard nicely-being

Decreased functionality to function in every day existence

Social isolation and stigma

It is important to word that possession is an tremendous incidence and can have underlying highbrow or scientific reasons. If you or someone you know is experiencing symptoms of ownership, it is crucial to are looking for for professional assist from an authorized healthcare professional or religious marketing consultant. Additionally, operating in the direction of right psychic protection strategies, consisting of grounding, visualization, and power protecting, can assist to save you ownership and sell stylish spiritual and psychic properly-being.

Generational Psychics

Generational psychics, moreover called familial or ancestral psychics, are humans who have inherited psychic talents or spiritual presents from previous generations of their circle of relatives. These competencies are believed to be exceeded down via genetics or spiritual lineage, and may show up in masses of strategies, together with clairvoyance, mediumship, recuperation, or divination.

Some examples of generational psychics embody:

Sylvia Browne: A famous psychic and creator, Sylvia Browne claimed to have inherited her psychic talents from her mom and grandmother. She became seemed for her art work as a medium, in addition to her psychic readings and appearances on television.

John Edward: Another famous medium and psychic, John Edward claimed to have inherited his gives from his mom and grandmother. He has written severa books near mediumship and psychic abilities, and has seemed on severa tv suggests.

Lisa Williams: A psychic and medium, Lisa Williams has claimed that her gifts had been handed down via her grandmother and excellent-grandmother. She has written numerous books on psychic improvement and has appeared on tv suggests consisting of "Lisa Williams: Life Among the Dead" and "Voices from the Other Side."

James Van Praagh: A medium and psychic, James Van Praagh has claimed that his items had been exceeded down from his grandmother, who emerge as also a medium. He has written several books on mediumship and spiritual improvement, and has seemed on television indicates collectively with "The Oprah Winfrey Show" and "Larry King Live."

Matt Fraser: A psychic medium and author, Matt Fraser claims to have inherited his items from his mother and grandmother. He is thought for his accuracy and has seemed on severa television shows and media shops.

Generational psychics can also art work with their ancestral lineage to tap into ancestral data and recovery energy, or to assist others hook up with their private ancestral lineage. They may additionally have a deeper understanding of their very very very own psychic skills and the way to expand them via their family information and spiritual lineage.

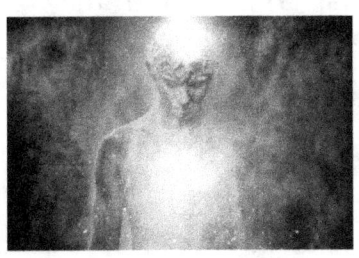

Chapter 4: The Bridge Between The Psychic And The Veil

The bridge the diverse psychic and the veil refers to the relationship among the bodily international and the spiritual realm. The "veil" is a time period used to offer an explanation for the separation many of the ones nation-states. For psychics, the capability to bridge the distance among the ones geographical regions lets in them to get right of access to statistics and insights which may be beyond the bodily international.

The veil is idea to be a barrier that separates the bodily global from the religious international. This barrier may be lifted or thinned via severa technique, collectively with via meditation, prayer, or the use of psychic tools like crystals, tarot playing cards, or pendulums. When the veil is thinned or lifted, it's miles believed that a psychic can greater outcomes get right of access to statistics from the religious realm.

Psychics who're capable of bridge the gap the various physical and religious geographical regions may additionally moreover experience lots of psychic phenomena, which includes clairvoyance (seeing beyond the physical realm), clairaudience (listening to past the physical realm), or clairsentience (sensing beyond the physical realm). These capabilities can be used to provide steering, restoration, or perception to others.

It is essential to phrase that the concept of the veil and the bridge many of the psychic and spiritual geographical areas may additionally variety amongst one-of-a-kind non secular and cultural traditions. Some can also view the veil as a eternal separation, at the same time as others may also see it as some thing that can be in brief lifted or thinned through specific practices or rituals. Nonetheless, the idea of the bridge among the psychic and the veil remains a treasured idea in hundreds of psychic and spiritual practices.

Best Psychic Crystals Needed for Development

Crystals are believed to maintain particular energies and vibrations that can be used to beautify psychic development. Here are a number of the great crystals for psychic development:

Amethyst - A famous crystal for psychic improvement, amethyst is thought to decorate intuition and religious attention. It is also said to protect in the direction of bad energies and promote a experience of calm.

Clear Quartz - Known because of the truth the "hold close healer" crystal, smooth quartz is believed to enlarge psychic abilities and beautify spiritual recognition. It is also stated to facilitate communique with higher nation-states.

Selenite - Selenite is a excessive-vibration crystal that is believed to enhance psychic talents, in particular clairvoyance and intuition. It is likewise stated to cleanse and purify the air of thriller.

Labradorite - Labradorite is perception to decorate psychic skills and instinct, particularly clairvoyance and telepathy. It is likewise said to shield in opposition to terrible energies and beautify religious increase.

Lapis Lazuli - Lapis lazuli is assumed to decorate psychic abilities and intuition, particularly clairvoyance and divination. It is also said to sell internal peace and religious hobby.

Fluorite - Fluorite is concept to beautify psychic abilities and instinct, particularly clairvoyance and telepathy. It is likewise stated to sell highbrow clarity and spiritual growth.

Black Tourmaline - Black tourmaline is notion to defend towards awful energies and psychic assault, making it a useful crystal for psychic improvement. It is likewise stated to promote grounding and a feel of stability.

It's crucial to phrase that on the equal time as crystals may be useful tools in psychic development, they are no longer a substitute for correct education and exercising. It's additionally critical to choose out crystals that resonate with you in my view, as every person's power is precise and can respond otherwise to taken into consideration one in every of a kind crystals.

Best uncommon crystals desired

While there are various commonly used crystals for psychic improvement, there also are some unusual and lesser-regarded crystals that can be enormously beneficial. Here are a few examples:

Phenacite - Phenacite is a rare crystal this is believed to enhance psychic abilities, specifically clairvoyance and non secular verbal exchange. It is also said to stimulate the 1/three eye chakra and promote spiritual boom.

Herkimer Diamond - Herkimer diamonds are a kind of double-terminated quartz crystal decided handiest in unique locations in New York u . S . A .. They are believed to decorate psychic abilities, especially clairvoyance and telepathy. They also are stated to promote non secular interest and reference to higher geographical regions.

Tanzanite - Tanzanite is a unprecedented blue-violet crystal that is believed to enhance psychic skills, especially clairvoyance and psychic vision. It is likewise stated to sell religious growth and connection with the better self.

Moldavite - Moldavite is a rare green crystal that is believed to beautify psychic skills, mainly clairvoyance and spiritual communique. It is likewise stated to stimulate the 1/three eye and crown chakras and promote spiritual increase.

Lemurian Seed Crystals - Lemurian seed crystals are unusual quartz crystals with precise ladder-like striations on their aspects.

They are believed to enhance psychic talents, in particular clairvoyance and spiritual verbal exchange. They are also said to keep the data and energy of the ancient civilization of Lemuria.

It's important to word that uncommon crystals can be extra hard to locate and may be more expensive than extra commonplace crystals. Additionally, it's miles vital to artwork with unusual crystals responsibly and ethically, ensuring that they may be sourced sustainably and with respect for the earth.

ASTROLOGY

Here's a listing of some of the primary astrological ideals and their cultures:

Western Astrology: The most generally recounted form of astrology, that is primarily based on the 12 zodiac signs and signs and symptoms and the vicinity of the planets on the time of a person's shipping. This way of life has roots in historical Babylonian and Egyptian astrology.

Chinese Astrology: This device is based totally definitely totally on a 12-3 hundred and sixty five days cycle of animal symptoms and signs and symptoms and signs and symptoms and signs and symptoms, with each yr being related to a completely precise animal. The Chinese zodiac is likewise related to the five elements of wooden, hearth, earth, steel, and water.

Vedic Astrology: Also referred to as Jyotish, this form of astrology comes from historic India and is based on the placement of the celebrities and planets on the time of a person's begin. Vedic astrology moreover takes under attention the lunar nodes, or Rahu and Ketu.

Mayan Astrology: This device is based on the Mayan calendar and is break up into 20 day symptoms, every with its very very personal particular this means that. The Mayans furthermore had a gadget of 13 numbers, which corresponded with the thirteen cycles of the moon.

Egyptian Astrology: This historical machine is based totally at the location of the celebs on the time of someone's delivery and is split into 12 symptoms, each related to a particular god or goddess.

Native American Astrology: Many Native American tribes had their very personal systems of astrology, often based totally mostly on the herbal cycles of the earth and the celebs. Some tribes associated wonderful animals with taken into consideration certainly one of a kind symptoms and believed that those animals had spiritual importance.

Tibetan Astrology: This device is based totally definitely mostly on the place of the celebs at the time of someone's start and is utilized in Tibet, Bhutan, and Nepal. It is similar to Vedic astrology, however furthermore consists of elements of Chinese astrology.

Arabic and Islamic Astrology: This system is primarily based on the teachings of ancient Greek philosophers and have become advanced within the route of the Islamic Golden Age. It includes both horoscopic astrology, based totally on the placement of the planets, and electional astrology, this is used to determine the amazing time to adopt fine movements.

Babylonian Astrology: One of the earliest identified structures of astrology, Babylonian astrology is based absolutely totally on the area of the planets at the time of someone's transport. The Babylonians also had a device of omens, which had been used to are anticipating destiny occasions

Now-

Let's open up approximately the western zodiac and list each astrological signal and their pleasant-appeared psychic developments

Aries (March 21 - April 19) - Aries is concept for their instinct and capability to feel the emotions of others.

Taurus (April 20 - May 20) - Taurus is perception for his or her capability to connect to nature and the earth's energies, further to their robust psychic protection.

Gemini (May 21 - June 20) - Gemini is understood for their telepathic abilities and functionality to read body language and subtle cues.

Cancer (June 21 - July 22) - Cancer is known for his or her sturdy empathic talents and capability to sense the emotions of others.

Leo (July 23 - August 22) - Leo is understood for their functionality to project their electricity and take location their dreams thru visualization.

Virgo (August 23 - September 22) - Virgo is concept for his or her capacity to revel in and study power patterns, in addition to their herbal recuperation abilties.

Libra (September 23 - October 22) - Libra is idea for his or her functionality to sense and stability energies, further to their functionality to examine auras.

Scorpio (October 23 - November 21) - Scorpio is thought for their strong psychic and intuitive abilities, specially within the areas of clairvoyance and psychometry.

Sagittarius (November 22 - December 21) - Sagittarius is understood for their capability to tap into better understanding and religious information.

Capricorn (December 22 - January 19) - Capricorn is understood for his or her capacity to seem their dreams and desires thru targeted purpose and practical motion.

Aquarius (January 20 - February 18) - Aquarius is belief for his or her functionality to connect with the collective attention and tap into ordinary expertise.

Pisces (February 19 - March 20) - Pisces is thought for his or her sturdy intuitive and psychic skills, especially inside the regions of clairvoyance and religious verbal exchange.

NATAL CHARTS and HOUSE PLACEMENTS

now we may want to speak about natal chart their house and the proper use of a natal chart

A natal chart, furthermore referred to as a beginning chart, is a image of the sky at the time of a person's starting. It provides notion into an person's personality, strengths, weaknesses, and existence direction. A natal chart is commonly divided into twelve sections, known as houses. Each residence is related to particular areas of lifestyles and can provide perception into considered one of a kind elements of a person's character and existence route.

Here is a quick compare of each house and its associated regions of existence:

1st House - The Self: This residence represents the person's personality, physical appearance, and technique to lifestyles.

2d House - Personal Finances: This house represents the individual's monetary scenario, private values, and material possessions.

0.33 House - Communication: This residence represents communique, mastering, and intellectual hobbies.

4th House - Home and Family: This house represents the man or woman's own family, childhood, and enjoy of protection.

fifth House - Creativity and Romance: This residence represents creativity, self-expression, romance, and kids.

6th House - Health and Work: This house represents the individual's bodily and intellectual fitness, every day sporting activities, and art work surroundings.

7th House - Relationships: This residence represents the individual's partnerships, marriage, and industrial employer relationships.

eighth House - Transformation: This house represents dying, rebirth, transformation, and shared sources.

ninth House - Travel and Higher Education: This residence represents tour, higher training, and non secular growth.

tenth House - Career: This residence represents the person's career, social recognition, and recognition.

11th House - Community: This house represents friendships, social organizations, and humanitarian motives.

12th House - Spirituality and Subconscious: This residence represents spirituality, goals, and the subconscious thoughts.

To properly use a natal chart, it's miles vital to have a fundamental expertise of astrology and the due to this of each house and planetary placement. A natal chart may be used as a device for self-interest and private increase, assisting individuals to understand their strengths, weaknesses, and lifestyles course. It can also offer notion into unique areas of existence, which incorporates career, relationships, and health.

One manner to use a natal chart is to find out the dominant planets and signs and symptoms in the chart, which could offer perception into the individual's character and dispositions. For example, someone with a dominant Mars can be assertive and motion-oriented, even as a person with a dominant Venus may be focused on relationships and aesthetics.

Another way to use a natal chart is to emerge as aware of any difficult elements or styles, along with a stellium (a interest of planets in a unmarried sign or residence) or a hard element among planets. These patterns can imply regions of life that can require greater hobby or strive to triumph over traumatic conditions and advantage non-public boom.

Overall, a natal chart can be a valuable device for self-discovery and private growth, imparting perception into an character's particular strengths, weaknesses, and lifestyles direction.

Babylonian Astrology -

Babylonian astrology, also known as Chaldean astrology, changed into one of the earliest types of astrology. It originated in historic Mesopotamia, now called Iraq, and have become practiced by using manner of the Babylonians and the Chaldeans.

The Babylonian zodiac consists of 12 symptoms and signs and symptoms and signs and symptoms and symptoms, each named after a constellation that come to be first-rate at some stage in a awesome time of the one year. The symptoms and their corresponding dates are:

MUL.APIN (The Plough) - March 21 to April 19

MUL.BABBAR (The Hired Man) - April 20 to May 20

MUL.SIPA.ZI.AN.NA (The Bull of Heaven) - May 21 to June 20

MUL.MUL (The Twins) - June 21 to July 22

MUL.LUGAL (The Crab) - July 23 to August 22

MUL.UR.GU.LA (The Lion) - August 23 to September 22

MUL.AB.SIN (The Scales) - September 23 to October 22

MUL.KAK.SI.SA (The Scorpion) - October 23 to November 21

MUL.GIR.TAB (The Archer) - November 22 to December 21

MUL.SUHUR.MASH (The Goat-Fish) - December 22 to January 19

MUL.AZAG.GI.INANA (The Water-Carrier) - January 20 to February 18

MUL.PA.BIL.SAG (The Fish-Goat) - February 19 to March 20

Each sign end up related to a ruling planet or celestial body, and every had its very non-public particular traits and symbolism. Babylonian astrology additionally positioned notable emphasis on the position and moves of the moon, as it changed into believed to have a effective have an effect on on human behavior and feelings.

Overall, Babylonian astrology became deeply ingrained inside the manner of lifestyles and society of ancient Mesopotamia, and its have an effect on can nevertheless be visible in present day astrology nowadays.

Now permit's open up on Mayan astrology and a way to use their chart system

Mayan astrology is an historical device of astrology that originated in Mesoamerica, and it's miles based totally completely on the Mayan calendar, that is a complicated tool of cycles and calendars that have been utilized by the Mayan civilization. Mayan astrology uses a one among a type device of astrology than Western astrology, with one-of-a-kind symbols and meanings.

The Mayan astrological chart is referred to as the Tzolkin, because of this "preserve in thoughts of days" within the Mayan language. The Tzolkin is a 260-day calendar that is made of 13-day cycles and 20 unique symbols or day signs and symptoms. Each day signal has its personal unique personality traits and traits, and every day within the Tzolkin has a selected strength and motive.

To use the Mayan astrological chart, you first need to decide your day signal, that is primarily based completely in your date of starting. The Mayan calendar has 20-day symptoms, which can be:

Imix

Ik

Akbal

Kan

Chicchan

Cimi

Manik

Lamat

Muluc

Oc

Chuen

Eb

Ben

Ix

Men

Cib

Caban

Etznab

Cauac

Ahau

Each day signal has its very very own set of persona inclinations, strengths, and weaknesses. For example, Imix is associated with introduction, instinct, and emotional intelligence, on the equal time as Ahau is associated with facts, control, and non secular increase.

Once you recognize your day signal, you could use the Tzolkin to decide your Mayan astrological chart. The Tzolkin is split into 20 rows, each of which represents a notable day sign. Each row is similarly divided into 13 columns, representing the thirteen-day cycles.

To create your Mayan astrological chart, you may need to discover your day sign inside the first row of the Tzolkin, and then be counted thirteen days to the right to discover your second day sign. You will maintain this system until you've got got got created a chart that is thirteen columns substantial and 20 rows prolonged.

Each column for your Mayan astrological chart represents a completely specific strength or topic, and every row represents a unique day signal. By analyzing your chart, you can benefit insight into your man or woman, strengths, weaknesses, and lifestyles path.

Mayan astrology is a complicated and complicated tool of astrology that calls for a deep statistics of the Mayan calendar and symbolism. However, with practice and examine, you can use the Mayan astrological chart to benefit belief into your individual and life route, and to assist manual you to your spiritual adventure.

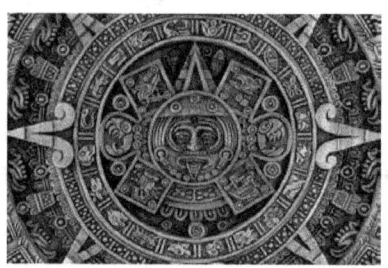

Tibetan Astrology-

Tibetan astrology, furthermore referred to as Tibetan cosmic generation, is a complex gadget of divination that dates another time to ancient times. It is based totally completely at the concepts of Buddhism and the lunar calendar, and it is believed to offer notion into one's man or woman, destiny, and fortune. The Tibetan astrological device includes twelve animal symptoms and signs and signs and symptoms and signs, 5 elements, and 8 trigrams.

Here is a breakdown of the twelve animal symptoms and signs and symptoms and signs and symptoms and signs and their corresponding years:

Rat: 1924, 1936, 1948, 1960, 1972, 1984, 1996, 2008, 2020

Ox: 1925, 1937, 1949, 1961, 1973, 1985, 1997, 2009, 2021

Tiger: 1926, 1938, 1950, 1962, 1974, 1986, 1998, 2010, 2022

Rabbit: 1927, 1939, 1951, 1963, 1975, 1987, 1999, 2011, 2023

Dragon: 1928, 1940, 1952, 1964, 1976, 1988, 2000, 2012, 2024

Snake: 1929, 1941, 1953, 1965, 1977, 1989, 2001, 2013, 2025

Horse: 1930, 1942, 1954, 1966, 1978, 1990, 2002, 2014, 2026

Sheep: 1931, 1943, 1955, 1967, 1979, 1991, 2003, 2015, 2027

Monkey: 1932, 1944, 1956, 1968, 1980, 1992, 2004, 2016, 2028

Rooster: 1933, 1945, 1957, 1969, 1981, 1993, 2005, 2017, 2029

Dog: 1934, 1946, 1958, 1970, 1982, 1994, 2006, 2018, 2030

Pig: 1935, 1947, 1959, 1971, 1983, 1995, 2007, 2019, 2031

In Tibetan astrology, every animal signal is associated with one of the 5 factors: earth, water, hearth, wood, or metal. The factors are believed to steer the personality and conduct of the man or woman born underneath that sign. Additionally, every animal signal is also related to one of the 8 trigrams, which represent the essential energies of the universe.

Tibetan astrology is commonly used for divination and to determine auspicious times for essential events, along with weddings and business enterprise gives. It is also believed to offer steering on one's spiritual course and can be used to determine compatibility amongst humans primarily based on their astrological charts.

Let's open up on Chinese zodiac

The Chinese zodiac is a device of astrology that has been used in China for over 2,000 years. It is based totally totally totally on a 12-yr cycle, with every twelve months associated with a first-rate animal signal. The 12 animal signs and symptoms and signs and symptoms and symptoms are: Rat, Ox, Tiger, Rabbit, Dragon, Snake, Horse, Goat, Monkey, Rooster, Dog, and Pig.

Each animal sign has its very own particular tendencies and individual traits, which might be stated to influence the individual born in that 12 months. Here is a short precis of the persona tendencies associated with every Chinese zodiac animal:

Rat: Quick-witted, progressive, bendy, and sort-hearted.

Ox: Diligent, dependable, strong, and decided.

Tiger: Brave, confident, competitive, and unpredictable.

Rabbit: Gentle, sensitive, considerate, and cautious.

Dragon: Confident, passionate, charismatic, and formidable.

Snake: Wise, mysterious, intuitive, and fashionable.

Horse: Adaptable, dependable, courageous, and ambitious.

Goat: Gentle, modern, clever, and peaceful.

Monkey: Clever, witty, curious, and playful.

Rooster: Honest, tough-going for walks, confident, and flamboyant.

Dog: Loyal, devoted, honest, and protecting.

Pig: Honest, kind, mild, and dependable.

In addition to the 12 animal symptoms and symptoms, the Chinese zodiac moreover has a 60-12 months cycle, which is manufactured from 12 animal signs and signs and five factors: Wood, Fire, Earth, Metal, and Water. Each mixture of animal sign and element is stated to have its very own specific strength and effect.

To determine your Chinese zodiac sign, you want to apprehend your start year. For instance, when you have been born in 1990, your Chinese zodiac signal might be the Horse. Once you apprehend your Chinese zodiac signal, you may examine greater about your individual tendencies and life direction based definitely mostly on the trends related to your sign.

The Chinese zodiac is a charming system of astrology that may provide insight into your individual and lifestyles course. By getting to know greater about your Chinese zodiac signal and the dispositions associated with it, you can advantage a deeper facts of yourself and those around you.

Arabic and Islamic Astrology-

It is a fusion of the Greek, Persian, and Indian traditions of astrology, and it's far been pretty influential inside the Islamic global and beyond. Here is a breakdown of Arabic and Islamic astrology and their signs and symptoms and signs and symptoms:

The 12 Signs:

The 12 signs and symptoms of Arabic and Islamic astrology are just like those of Western astrology, but with Arabic names. The signs, in order, are:

Aries: Al Hamal

Taurus: Al Thurayya

Gemini: Al Jawza

Cancer: Al Saratan

Leo: Al Asad

Virgo: Al Sunbula

Libra: Al Mizan

Scorpio: Al 'Aqrab

Sagittarius: Al Qaws

Capricorn: Al Jadi

Aquarius: Al Dalw

Pisces: Al Hût

The Planets:

Arabic and Islamic astrology makes use of the equal seven planets as Western astrology, but with some versions in interpretation. The planets, so as of distance from the Earth, are:

Saturn: Zuhal

Jupiter: Mushtari

Mars: Marikh

Sun: Shams

Venus: Zuhra

Mercury: Utarid

Moon: Qamar

The Houses:

The Arabic and Islamic astrological homes are the same as those of Western astrology, however they're traditionally numbered in opposite order, from 12 to at least one. Each house is associated with a particular region of lifestyles and has a ruling planet.

The Lunar Mansions:

Arabic and Islamic astrology additionally makes use of the lunar mansions, or stations, which can be primarily based definitely on the ranges of the Moon. There are 28 lunar mansions, each associated with a particular celebrity or constellation.

Interpretation:

Arabic and Islamic astrology places exquisite emphasis on the place of fate and the have an effect on of the celebrities and planets on human destiny. The horoscope is used to offer steering and belief into all areas of lifestyles, together with relationships, career, fitness, and spirituality.

In give up, Arabic and Islamic astrology is a rich and complicated device that has been especially influential within the Islamic worldwide and past. It stocks many similarities with Western astrology however also has some precise functions, consisting of the usage of Arabic names for the signs and symptoms and symptoms and planets and the emphasis on fate and destiny.

Vedic astrology

Vedic astrology is a machine of astrology that originated in historical India and has been practiced for over five,000 years. It is also known as Jyotish, which means that that "era of mild" in Sanskrit. Vedic astrology is based totally at the sidereal zodiac, which takes into consideration the constant stars within the sky, similarly to the actions of the planets.

The basis of Vedic astrology is the concept of karma, which holds that our moves and thoughts in this life and previous lives create a pattern of strength that influences our future. The purpose of Vedic astrology is to assist human beings understand their karmic patterns and make alternatives that align with their most purpose.

Vedic astrology uses a complicated system of calculations to create a beginning chart, it honestly is a map of the positions of the planets on the time of an man or woman's start. This start chart is used to advantage belief into the person's persona, relationships, profession, and life route.

The Vedic begin chart is break up into 12 houses, every of which represents a selected detail of lifestyles, which incorporates fitness, fee variety, and relationships. Each house is likewise associated with a ruling planet, that may affect the power of that house.

Vedic astrology additionally makes use of a machine of planetary periods, called dashas, which advise the intervals of time even as unique planets are most influential in an character's life. These dashas are used to make predictions and provide steerage on the way to navigate fantastic periods of life.

Vedic astrology is a complicated and nuanced machine of astrology that could provide deep insights into an person's lifestyles path and motive. By records the patterns and energies of the planets and the homes of their beginning chart, human beings can make extra informed picks and navigate their lives with more readability and reason.

Egyptian Zodiac-

There are 12 symptoms and signs inside the Egyptian zodiac, every corresponding to a one-of-a-type month of the 12 months. Here is a breakdown of the signs and their meanings:

The Nile (Jan 1-7, Jun 19-28, Sep 1-7, Nov 18-26): Those born below the Nile sign are stated to be revolutionary, intelligent, and natural leaders. They are also identified for their adaptability and resilience.

Amon-Ra (Jan eight-21, Feb 1-eleven): Those born beneath the Amon-Ra sign are stated to be confident, ambitious, and passionate. They are herbal leaders who are not afraid to take risks.

Mut (Jan 22-31, Sep eight-22): Those born under the Mut sign are stated to be nurturing, shielding, and compassionate. They are frequently seen because the caretakers in their groups.

Geb (Feb 12-29, Aug 20-31): Those born underneath the Geb sign are said to be sensible, hardworking, and down-to-earth. They are also recounted for their humorousness and their love of nature.

Osiris (Mar 1-10, Nov 27-Dec 18): Those born below the Osiris sign are said to be sturdy-willed, independent, and progressive. They are often visible as rebels who undertaking authority.

Isis (Mar eleven-31, Oct 18-29, Dec 19-31): Those born underneath the Isis sign are stated to be compassionate, nurturing, and intuitive. They are also recognized for his or her robust intuition and their capability to heal others.

Thoth (Apr 1-19, Nov eight-17): Those born beneath the Thoth signal are said to be smart, curious, and analytical. They are herbal trouble solvers who aren't afraid to tackle complicated disturbing situations.

Horus (Apr 20-May 7, Aug 12-19): Those born underneath the Horus signal are said to be confident, ambitious, and decided. They are herbal leaders who aren't afraid to take risks.

Anubis (May 8-27, Jun 29-Jul 13): Those born underneath the Anubis sign are stated to be impartial, innovative, and mysterious. They are frequently visible due to the fact the guardians of secrets and techniques.

Seth (May 28-Jun 18, Sep 28-Oct 2, Nov 27-Dec 18): Those born under the Seth sign are said to be ambitious, assured, and decided. They are natural leaders who aren't afraid to take risks.

Bastet (Jul 14-28, Sep 23-27, Oct three-17): Those born beneath the Bastet sign are stated to be independent, innovative, and charismatic. They are often visible due to the fact the life of the birthday celebration.

Sekhmet (Jul 29-Aug eleven, Oct 30-Nov 7): Those born under the Sekhmet sign are stated to be powerful, passionate, and extreme. They are often visible because the protectors of their groups.

Native American Astrology –

Native American astrology is based totally on the perception that everybody has an animal totem that guides and impacts their person tendencies and existence path. These totems are represented with the beneficial resource of various animals, and every animal has its private specific developments and traits. Here is a breakdown of the Native American zodiac signs and symptoms and signs and their meanings:

Otter (January 20 - February 18): Otter human beings are mentioned for their playful and curious nature. They are revolutionary, realistic, and often have a completely unique angle on the world.

Wolf (February 19 - March 20): Wolf human beings are intuitive, emotional, and deeply associated with their religious issue. They are natural healers and feature a sturdy revel in of empathy.

Falcon (March 21 - April 19): Falcon humans are ambitious, pushed, and constantly seeking out new disturbing conditions. They are natural leaders and function a robust enjoy of self-self assurance.

Beaver (April 20 - May 20): Beaver people are hardworking, practical, and dependable. They are professional at constructing and developing subjects, and often have a strong connection to the earth.

Deer (May 21 - June 20): Deer people are curious, adaptable, and feature a love for getting to know. They are frequently fantastic communicators and characteristic a natural capacity to hook up with others.

Chapter 5: Sigils

Sigils are symbols which may be used in magic and occult practices to symbolize a selected goal or choice. They are created with the aid of way of mixing unique symbols, letters, and shapes in a totally particular manner to create a visible instance of the practitioner's aim.

The machine of creating a sigil is typically carried out thru a way of meditation or visualization, in which the practitioner makes a speciality of their motive after which creates a photograph that represents that cause. This photo is then charged with strength and utilized in quite a few methods, together with in spells, rituals, or as a talisman for protection or manifestation.

One of the most not unusual techniques of creating a sigil is thru a manner called "sigilization." This consists of writing out the goal or desire in a sentence, and then doing away with all repeating letters and vowels. The last letters are then blended and rearranged into a very unique photo that represents the aim.

Sigils may be utilized in quite a few procedures, counting on the aim of the practitioner. For instance, they'll be inscribed on candles, drawn on paper or material, or maybe tattooed onto the pores and skin. They also can be utilized in aggregate with notable magical practices, which include meditation or ritual, to extend their strength and effectiveness.

Overall, sigils are a powerful tool for practitioners of magic and the occult, as they allow for the manifestation of specific intentions and dreams in a seen and tangible manner.

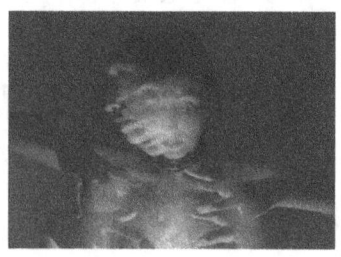

NDE and Astral Projection

NDE (Near-Death Experience) and Astral Projection are phenomena that are often related to heightened levels of psychic popularity.

Near-Death Experience happens whilst an character comes near loss of lifestyles or is clinically dead for a brief time body after which revived. During this time, the man or woman may also enjoy numerous psychic phenomena, at the facet of seeing incredible lighting fixtures, feeling a experience of peace or detachment from the frame, encountering deceased loved ones or non secular beings, and gaining new insights or views on life.

Astral Projection, however, is a exercise in which an character deliberately separates their consciousness from their physical frame and travels out of doors of it. This may be achieved thru meditation, lucid dreaming, or one-of-a-type strategies. During astral projection, human beings might also experience numerous psychic phenomena, together with seeing their personal body from a notable perspective, encountering religious beings or entities, and gaining new insights or perspectives at the person of fact.

Both NDE and Astral Projection can be seen as examples of the manner heightened ranges of psychic interest can purpose critiques that go past normal waking attention. They provide a glimpse into the capability power of the human mind and the possibility of exploring top notch geographical regions of lifestyles beyond the physical international.

It is vital to have a take a look at that each NDE and Astral Projection also can be unstable practices, as they contain probably leaving the bodily body inside the lower back of and venturing into unknown or probably risky territories. It is commonly endorsed that folks who are interested in exploring those practices achieve this under the steering of skilled instructors or practitioners, and with a robust foundation in psychic safety and grounding strategies.

Near-Death Experiences (NDE)

Near-Death Experiences (NDE) are profound and transformative memories that would occur while someone is on the brink of lack of life or has been declared clinically useless however is later revived. These tales were suggested during cultures and within the path of records and frequently comprise a whole lot of psychic and mystical memories.

During an NDE, human beings document a experience of leaving their bodily frame and entering a brand new, otherworldly realm. They regularly describe feelings of peace, love, and interconnectedness, in addition to encounters with religious beings, deceased loved ones, and a effective, loving presence that is regularly interpreted as God or the divine.

Psychic skills are also frequently stated during NDEs, at the facet of telepathy, clairvoyance, precognition, and heightened intuition. Many humans record receiving profound insights and steerage that assist them to recognize their life reason and the character of truth.

While NDEs are often transformative and lifestyles-converting, they also may be tough to mix into one's everyday existence. It is critical to are seeking out guide from relied on specialists, including counselors or non secular advisors, to help method those evaluations and integrate them into one's non-public ideals and values.

ONE Astral Projection

Astral Projection, additionally known as out-of-body reports (OBE), is the enjoy of preserving apart one's recognition from the physical frame and journeying in an astral or energy body to other dimensions or places. This is a phenomenon that has been said all through history and in the course of cultures.

Astral Projection is frequently skilled spontaneously or caused through meditation, lucid dreaming, or precise altered states of cognizance. It is stated to be a natural psychic potential that can be evolved with exercise and schooling.

During an astral projection, human beings file quite loads of psychic reviews, which includes telepathy, clairvoyance, and precognition. They additionally document encounters with religious beings, deceased cherished ones, and different entities in superb dimensions or parallel realities.

One of the blessings of astral projection is the capacity to advantage insights and information that aren't available inside the physical worldwide. This includes a deeper understanding of one's lifestyles motive, the person of truth, and non secular truths.

However, it's miles important to technique astral projection with warning and respect. It is crucial to floor oneself in advance than and after the enjoy, to set intentions and guard oneself from bad energies or entities, and to searching for guidance from skilled practitioners or teachers. It is also crucial to be aware of the functionality risks, collectively with the possibility of turning into out of place or disoriented in a single-of-a-kind dimensions or being no longer capable of return to the bodily frame.

NDE information approximately the claims of the spirit realm

Near-lack of life memories (NDEs) are often said via human beings who have been clinically dead or close to lack of lifestyles and then revived. Many who revel in NDEs record comparable capabilities together with a feeling of separation from their body, a experience of peace and calm, and the perception of being in a spiritual realm. Here are some of the generally stated records approximately the spirit realm in NDEs:

A feeling of peace and quietness: Many humans file feeling a sense of peace and quietness when they enter the spirit realm. This feeling may be overwhelming and is often defined as being within the presence of a loving being.

A revel in of timelessness: Time is regularly said as being distorted or non-existent inside the spirit realm. Many humans document feeling like they were there for only a few mins, however in truth, hours may moreover have exceeded.

Meeting loved ones who have exceeded away: Many humans document seeing and interacting with cherished ones who've surpassed away. This may be a comforting enjoy for those who've misplaced someone close to them.

Life assessment: Many human beings report experiencing a existence examine wherein they see their lifestyles flash earlier than their eyes. This is often defined as being a non-judgmental experience where the man or woman sees their lifestyles from a brand new thoughts-set.

Seeing a moderate: Many people document seeing a vibrant moderate or being drawn inside the direction of a mild source within the spirit realm. This light is frequently defined as being heat and alluring.

Being in a considered one of a type size: Many humans file feeling like they have got entered a unique size or truth after they input the spirit realm. This may be hard to provide an explanation for, however it is regularly stated as feeling like a certainly one of a kind diploma of lifestyles.

It is critical to word that even as those studies are not unusual, no longer truely everybody who has an NDE reviews the equal competencies. NDEs are pretty non-public reminiscences, and the specifics can range notably from character to character.

Psychic Abilities Can Save Lives

Psychic competencies, together with telepathy, clairvoyance, and intuition, may be worthwhile in supporting to preserve lives. There were severa bills of psychics who've used their abilties to warn others of chance or to provide crucial statistics in emergency conditions.

One instance is the case of Lori Palmer, a psychic who assisted inside the search for a lacking boy in California. Palmer had a imaginative and prescient of the boy's place and shared this records with the government. Her vision have end up out to be accurate, and the boy become located alive and nicely.

Another instance is the tale of Benny, a psychic dog who stored his owner's lifestyles. Benny have grow to be capable of feel that his owner emerge as in misery and ran to a nearby avenue to save you a passing automobile. The riding strain, who become a nurse, have become able to provide scientific help and speak to for an ambulance, in the long run saving the owner's lifestyles.

Psychic talents also can be beneficial in predicting and stopping disasters. For example, there have been reviews of psychics who have had premonitions about natural disasters, along with earthquakes or hurricanes, and were able to warn others in advance. This allows for evacuation and education, probably saving infinite lives.

Additionally, psychics can offer consolation and closure to households who've out of area cherished ones. They can be in a position to speak with spirits on the other factor and offer messages of love and reassurance. This can deliver a experience of peace to individuals who are grieving and help them to transport in advance in their recovery technique.

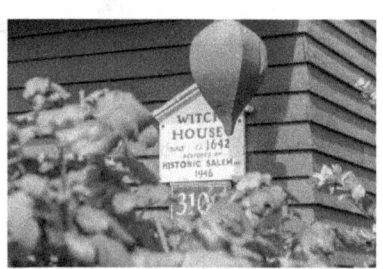

In quit, psychic competencies have the capacity to keep lives in a number of strategies. While they'll be tough to quantify or degree, there are various money owed of psychics the use of their affords to make a fine difference inside the global. As such, it's miles vital to technique psychic skills with an open thoughts and a willingness to find out their capacity for unique.

Chapter 6: Historical Psychic Oppression

Throughout facts, human beings with psychic competencies had been every revered and feared. Many historic cultures believed in the energy of psychics and may are looking for recommendation from them for steering on important subjects. However, with the upward push of prepared religion and medical rationalism, the credibility of psychic capabilities changed into known as into query. Despite this, there are various documented instances of humans with psychic abilities, collectively with clairvoyance, telekinesis, and telepathy.

In the 20 th century, governments across the place started out to take an hobby in psychic abilties, particularly as they related to country wide safety. During the Cold War, every the USA and the Soviet Union invested closely in psychic studies, hoping to gain a navy gain over their enemies. This added approximately the formation of applications which encompass the CIA's Project Stargate and the Soviet Union's Psi Corps.

These programs worried the usage of psychics to build up intelligence, conduct a long way off viewing operations, or even attempt to steer the mind and moves of others. While there may be a few proof that the ones packages produced results, they had been in the long run near down due to lack of proof and public scrutiny.

However, some take into account that the authorities keeps to suppress the improvement of psychic talents. This can be due to a fear that people with psychic skills have to disrupt the set up order, or because psychic competencies are visible as a risk to the strength of the ruling class.

Regardless of the reasons, there's a developing motion to encompass psychic abilties and to apply them for the advantage of all. Many people recollect that psychic talents have the functionality to shop lives, with the useful resource of supplying caution of drawing near failures or thru manner of supporting to find out lacking people.

There are many examples of people with psychic talents who have used their gadgets to help others. For example, inside the aftermath of the 2011 earthquake and tsunami in Japan, a girl named Hiromi Motohashi claimed that she had obtained a message from her deceased grandmother caution of the approaching catastrophe. She warned her pals and circle of relatives, and lots of had been able to evacuate in advance than the tsunami hit.

In each other case, a lady named Nancy Weber used her psychic capabilities to assist find lacking individuals. She worked with regulation enforcement businesses to offer statistics that helped discover numerous missing human beings, which incorporates a missing toddler who had been kidnapped.

While there can be but lots skepticism surrounding psychic competencies, there is moreover a growing popularity that they may be real and beneficial. As our knowledge of the human mind and focus maintains to evolve, it is feasible that we may additionally find out even more about the capability of psychic capabilities to keep lives and make the area a better area.

Nostradamus (surely one in every of my guides) became a French scientific physician, astrologer, and famend seer who lived at a few degree inside the 16th century. He acquired reputation for his prophetic works, which is probably stated to have efficaciously anticipated many fundamental worldwide activities, which includes the upward push of Napoleon Bonaparte, the French Revolution, and World War II.

In addition to his paintings as a seer, Nostradamus additionally served as a health practitioner to several individuals of the French royal court docket docket, which consist of Catherine de' Medici, the queen consort of King Henry II of France. It became via this function that Nostradamus received get right of entry to to essential political figures and modified into able to use his psychic competencies to offer precious insights into subjects of nation.

One of the maximum famous instances of Nostradamus' predictions being used inside the royal court docket docket concerned his prediction of the loss of life of King Henry II. Nostradamus reportedly warned the king of an coming near near chance, however his warnings went unheeded. On July 10, 1559, on the identical time as taking element in a jousting event, King Henry II modified into struck in the attention thru a lance and died from his accidents, fun Nostradamus' prophecy.

Nostradamus' accuracy in predicting destiny activities, combined alongside along with his position as a doctor to the royal court docket, made him a precious asset to the French monarchy. His predictions were carefully studied and taken into hobby with the useful aid of many members of the court, together with Queen Catherine, who became stated to be a strong believer in his capabilities.

However, his predictions have been additionally the situation of lots controversy and skepticism all through his lifetime, and stay debated via students and enthusiasts to in recent times.

As a psychic network, it is important to apprehend the records of oppression and suppression of our abilties, and to take preventative measures to make sure that it in no way takes vicinity another time. In the past, folks who exhibited psychic talents had been often visible as a risk to the ones in electricity, and have been therefore oppressed or perhaps persecuted. This has led to a cultural fear and rejection of psychic capabilities in lots of components of the sector.

In order to save you this from taking area over again, we ought to actively paintings to exchange the narrative surrounding psychic abilities. This approach coaching ourselves and others approximately the truth of psychic talents and their potential advantages, at the equal time as additionally acknowledging and addressing any dangerous beliefs or behaviors that can be contributing to their oppression.

Additionally, we need to art work to bring together a sturdy and supportive network of psychics who can offer a strong area for human beings with psychic competencies to increase and expand. This can encompass developing networks for sharing knowledge and assets, further to supplying emotional help and steerage to those who may be struggling with the demanding situations of dwelling with psychic talents.

Finally, it's miles crucial to recognize the location that religious and lively practices can play in maintaining and protecting our psychic abilities. By often working towards meditation, visualization, electricity artwork, and awesome strategies, we are able to enhance our connection to our psychic skills and domesticate a feel of inner strength and resilience that could help us to resist any tries to oppress or suppress our gives.

In short, with the useful aid of going for walks together as a community, instructing others, and actively protective and strengthening our abilities, we can prevent the oppression of psychics from ever taking area over again.

Higher Realm Education

Yes, there are real psychic colleges and complete-time paying jobs for humans with superior recognition.

Here are a few information on wherein to find out those opportunities and related charges:

Psychic Schools:

The Arthur Findlay College of Psychic Science inside the UK: This college offers a massive variety of guides on psychic development, mediumship, healing, and one of a kind associated subjects. The guides are taught by using the use of the usage of experienced psychic teachers and range in duration from subsequently to severa weeks. The value of courses varies counting on the period and state of affairs rely, but a one-week path can price around £500-£800.

The Rhine Research Center within the US: This middle gives some of publications on psychic phenomena and parapsychology. The publications range from one-day workshops to on-line publications and are taught with the resource of skilled researchers and teachers. The fee of guides varies counting on the length and scenario depend, however a one-day workshop can charge spherical $a hundred.

The Berkeley Psychic Institute in the US: This institute gives a complete application on psychic improvement, restoration, and communication. The software consists of 24 weeks of training and consists of lectures, bodily sports, and exercise periods. The rate of this tool is $1,800.

Full-Time Paying Jobs:

Psychic Reader: Many psychic readers work for psychic hotlines, online structures, or in-person psychic stores. The pay varies relying on the agency and the experience of the reader, however on common, psychic readers may want to make round $20-$30 in step with hour.

Psychic Investigator: Some police departments and personal research businesses hire psychic investigators to help with missing man or woman times and exclusive investigations. The pay varies relying on the business corporation and the revel in of the investigator, however on average, psychic investigators ought to make round $50-$100 in line with hour.

Psychic Medium: Some psychic mediums provide their services to clients for non-public readings, organization durations, or sports. The pay varies relying at the experience and recognition of the medium, but on not unusual, psychic mediums must make round $100-$two hundred in line with hour.

It's crucial to take a look at that the psychic employer isn't regulated, so it is vital to do studies and choose out proper schools and corporations to work with. Additionally, no longer all psychic abilties are monetizable or with out issues marketable, so it's crucial to technique psychic development with a balanced and down to earth thoughts-set.

Seeing is Believing

The Pineal Gland, additionally known as the "1/3 eye," is a small endocrine gland located within the mind. While it's miles a fairly small organ, it plays an critical characteristic in regulating our sleep and wake cycles, in addition to the secretion of melatonin, a hormone that enables us sleep. However, many human beings consider that the Pineal Gland has a much more reason beyond those easy functions.

One of the essential element elements which have been connected to the Pineal Gland is the production of N-dimethyltryptamine, or DMT. DMT is a powerful psychedelic compound that is produced in truth within the human frame, such as the Pineal Gland. It is frequently known as the "spirit molecule" because of its potential to prompt altered states of consciousness, together with mystical and spiritual reviews.

Many human beings don't forget that the Pineal Gland and DMT play a critical function in psychic attention. Some even advocate that the Pineal Gland is the bodily vicinity of the zero.33 eye and that its activation is important for superior psychic talents to appear.

While the concept of the Pineal Gland being the essential aspect to unlocking psychic abilties stays a depend of dialogue within the medical network, there are various practices that people can have interaction in to help activate the Pineal Gland and increase their psychic attention. One such exercise is breathwork.

Breathwork consists of intentionally controlling the breath to stimulate the frame's herbal rest response. This can motive a heightened country of recognition and an extended enjoy of connectedness to the arena round us. Breathwork also can help spark off the Pineal Gland and increase the producing of DMT.

Diet is likewise an vital detail in activating the Pineal Gland and developing psychic awareness. Some food which have been related to Pineal Gland activation consist of darkish leafy greens, end end result, nuts, and seeds. Additionally, fending off processed elements, alcohol, and caffeine can assist sell a wholesome Pineal Gland and accelerated psychic consciousness.

Sleep is some different crucial element in Pineal Gland feature and psychic awareness. Getting enough sleep and keeping a regular sleep time table can assist make sure that the Pineal Gland is functioning properly and that DMT manufacturing is pinnacle-pleasant.

Stress is every distinct element which could negatively effect Pineal Gland feature and psychic interest. Engaging in regular pressure-decreasing practices on the facet of meditation, yoga, or tai chi can assist lessen pressure tiers and sell healthful Pineal Gland function.

In precis, the Pineal Gland and its dating to DMT play a big feature in psychic attention. While the idea that the Pineal Gland is the bodily area of the zero.33 eye remains a recollect of dialogue, there are numerous practices together with breathwork, diet regime, sleep, and stress reduce charge that might help set off the Pineal Gland and boom psychic attention.

Spirit Molecules

DMT, or N,N-Dimethyltryptamine, is a powerful psychedelic compound that has been used for hundreds of years in conventional Amazonian shamanic practices. DMT can activate a profound altered united states of recognition, often defined as a "step forward" or "pinnacle" experience. Many human beings report encountering otherworldly entities or beings in the course of DMT trips.

The testimonies cautioned for the duration of DMT journeys variety considerably, however commonplace subjects include encounters with beings which might be often described as "tool elves," "aliens," or "entities." These beings might also additionally furthermore talk telepathically with the individual or impart expertise and knowledge.

There are severa theories as to why DMT can also bring about those studies. Some agree with that DMT reasons the discharge of endogenous DMT in the mind, that can supply an reason for the reviews of encounters with otherworldly beings. Others keep in mind that the reminiscences are in number one phrases subjective and are virtually a made from the man or woman's very personal psyche.

Regardless of the mechanism, DMT journeys can be a effective tool for exploring the man or woman of consciousness and the mysteries of the universe. However, it is important to method DMT use with caution and recognize. DMT is a effective substance which could activate immoderate reports, and it must best be used under the supervision of an experienced and informed practitioner.

Factors which consist of weight loss plan, sleep, and stress tiers can also impact the first rate of DMT reminiscences. Many customers document that following a healthy eating regimen and getting superb sufficient sleep can help prepare the thoughts and body for a DMT ride. Additionally, reducing strain and anxiety tiers can help to create a extra outstanding and effective thoughts-set for exploring the geographical regions of reputation.

In prevent, on the equal time as DMT trips may offer insights into the man or woman of reality and the universe, they want to be approached with caution and recognize. It is essential to put together the mind and frame thru practices along with breathwork, meditation, and wholesome way of life alternatives to make certain the nice possible experience.

DMT may be breath activated-

It is critical to phrase that DMT is a Schedule I managed substance in most international locations and it's far illegal to apply it for enjoyment features. However, some human beings use breathwork and meditation strategies to set off DMT genuinely of their brains.

Here are some steps which may be commonly advised for breathwork to set off DMT:

Find a quiet and comfortable area in which you won't be disturbed for at the least half-hour.

Sit in a snug characteristic at the side of your another time at once and your toes flat on the floor.

Begin via taking some deep breaths, inhaling via your nostril and exhaling through your mouth. Try to recognition in your breath and allow circulate of any distractions or thoughts.

Once you feel comfortable, begin to breathe inside and outside through your nose in a rhythmic pattern. The endorsed sample is to inhale for 4 seconds, hold your breath for seven seconds, and then exhale for eight seconds.

As you continue to breathe, attempt to visualize a colourful white mild getting into your body with each inhale and developing throughout your frame. With each exhale, visualize any awful energy or tension leaving your frame.

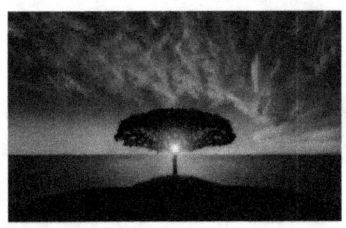

Keep inhaling this sample for at the least 15-20 minutes, or till you sense a revel in of clarity, euphoria, or special altered states of interest.

It is crucial to study that DMT breathwork should most effective be tried with the useful resource of the usage of skilled human beings and with caution. It is also important to keep in mind the ability risks and crook implications earlier than trying any strategies that incorporate the use of DMT.

Chapter 7: Astral Projection Guidelines

Astral projection is a manner that permits a person's cognizance to head away their bodily body and discover the astral plane. It may be a powerful tool for spiritual boom and exploration. Here are a few hints for beginners who need to strive astral projection:

Prepare your vicinity: Find a quiet, comfortable area wherein you may lighten up with out being disturbed. The room need to be darkish and quiet, and you want to experience constant and snug. You can also use candles, incense, or distinctive gadgets to help you create a peaceful and calming surroundings.

Relax your frame: Start through exciting your frame. Lie down in a comfortable feature and reputation to your breath. Take gradual, deep breaths and experience your frame begin to loosen up. You can also strive cutting-edge muscle relaxation, in that you traumatic and loosen up every muscle agency on your frame separately.

Focus your mind: Once your frame is relaxed, you may start to recognition your thoughts. Visualize yourself floating or flying, and believe your self leaving your physical frame. You can also repeat a mantra or attention on a selected item to help quiet your mind.

Enter the vibrational kingdom: As you start to sense extra cushty and centered, you may begin to revel in a humming or vibrating sensation in your body. This is an indication that you're entering into the vibrational country, it honestly is a precursor to astral projection. Focus on the sensation and attempt to stay comfortable.

Visualize your holiday spot: Once you're in the vibrational country, you can begin to visualize your excursion spot. Imagine yourself floating out of your frame and flying to a selected vicinity. You can also try to discover a portal or doorway on the way to take you to the astral aircraft.

Stay centered: It's crucial to live centered and comfortable in the course of the astral projection revel in. Don't allow your mind wander, and try no longer to get too excited or scared. If you begin to sense uncomfortable, you may constantly go lower back in your bodily body through clearly thinking about it.

Practice often: Astral projection takes exercising, so do no longer get discouraged in case you do not be successful right away. Try to exercising at the same time each day, and hold a mag to music your improvement. With time and exercising, you may amplify a deeper expertise of the astral plane and your own recognition.

spirit guides and a way to get to realise them

Spirit publications are non-physical beings who're believed to offer steerage, assist, and recognise-the way to the ones at the physical plane. They are now and again referred to as parent angels, religious courses, or genuinely publications.

Getting to comprehend your spirit courses requires an open mind and a willingness to talk with them. Here are some tips for connecting together along with your spirit publications:

Set your aim: The first step is to set your aim to hook up with your spirit publications. This may be finished via prayer, meditation, or really affirming your goal out loud.

Clear your thoughts: It's critical to easy your mind of any distractions and focus to your motive. Take a few deep breaths and permit your self to loosen up.

Ask for a sign: Ask your spirit guides to offer you a signal that they're gift. This may be a feel, a sensation, or a picture.

Trust your intuition: Pay hobby to any thoughts, feelings, or sensations that come to you. These can be messages out of your spirit publications.

Communicate collectively collectively along with your courses: Once you enjoy which you have made a connection with your spirit courses, ask them for steerage or recommendation. Listen to their responses and receive as actual collectively along with your intuition.

Practice often: Connecting along side your spirit guides is a capacity that takes exercise. Set aside time each day to meditate, pray, or definitely communicate in conjunction with your publications.

Remember, spirit guides are usually present and prepared to help. All you want to do is be open to their steerage and willing to pay attention.

Remember to Relax

Feeling on top of things with psychic competencies is an vital factor of developing and the use of them. Without manage, one can also come to be overwhelmed, disturbing, or even scared of their abilties, essential to a horrible effect on their bodily, emotional, and intellectual fitness. Therefore, it's far vital to understand the manner to take a destroy or quickly halt your psychic work if you sense like it is becoming an excessive amount of to deal with.

One of the number one steps in gaining control of your psychic talents is through meditation and grounding techniques. Regular meditation and grounding practices permit you to live centered, calm, and targeted, and similarly they offer you with the functionality to disconnect from your abilties while important. These strategies can embody respiration physical video games, visualization, and extraordinary rest strategies.

It is also crucial to set boundaries for your self and others. This manner knowledge and talking what you are and are not comfortable with with regards to your psychic skills. For example, you could no longer need to apply your talents to have a study someone's mind with out their permission, otherwise you couldn't want to use your talents at the same time as you feel emotionally unstable.

If you revel in like you need to take a wreck out of your psychic skills, there are various topics you can do. The first step is to renowned that you need a ruin and to no longer experience accountable about it. Taking a harm is a herbal and crucial part of psychic development, and it's miles crucial to honor your dreams and boundaries.

During your ruin, you may need to focus on self-care and rest strategies. This can embody getting enough sleep, eating nicely, and appealing in sports activities activities that make you revel in well, at the side of spending time with loved ones or accomplishing hobbies.

It is likewise critical to are looking for assist from others, such as a depended on pal or a expert therapist, if you are experiencing trouble coping with your competencies or feel beaten.

In precis, feeling on top of things of your psychic skills is critical to your ordinary properly-being. By growing grounding techniques, setting obstacles, and taking breaks, whilst critical, you may preserve a wholesome stability amongst using your competencies and taking care of your self.

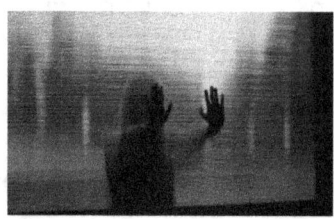

Spiritual Warfare and our Psychic Revolution

Spiritual war is a time period used to give an cause of the conflict amongst horrific entities and the psychic or person who is trying to defend themselves or others. It includes the usage of psychic gives and religious practices to combat towards terrible energies and entities that can be seeking to harm or own a person.

In non secular struggle, psychics use their abilties to find out and become aware of awful energies and entities that can be located in a specific space. They can also use gear like crystals, candles, or sage to create a protecting barrier and push back horrible energies.

The psychic may also moreover art work with a crew of other psychics or religious practitioners to perform a collective non secular cleansing and safety ritual. This can contain reciting prayers, chanting, or using particular non secular techniques to banish awful energies and entities. In trendy years it has been more of a trending records-remembering beyond lives and origins so firmly with psychic schooling that its sparking an upward push up of Alien help- actually and it's miles referred to as The Great Awakening and The Starseeds. (amongst numerous other titles, which have supported the psychic network)

The concept of Starseeds refers to people who have incarnated on Earth however originated from unique planets or film superstar structures in the universe. Many folks that grow to be aware about as Starseeds take delivery of as real with they very own psychic abilties because of their extraterrestrial beginning.

According to the Starseed idea, the ones people own a better degree of popularity and non secular awareness than the not unusual person due to their past lives on one-of-a-kind planets. They may additionally additionally have innate psychic competencies which incorporates telepathy, clairvoyance, or channeling, which they might use to connect with their extraterrestrial origins and result in effective trade on Earth.

Some Starseeds may additionally experience a sturdy experience of assignment or purpose on Earth, which may additionally include the use of their psychic talents to assist others or to promote spiritual increase and awakening.

They also can revel in a sturdy experience of connection to nature, animals, and special beings on Earth and inside the universe.

However, it's crucial to word that now not all psychics perceive as Starseeds, and no longer all Starseeds find out as psychics. While the 2 requirements may be related in some instances, they may be now not constantly collectively specific.

In any case, many folks that are interested in psychic improvement may additionally moreover furthermore find out concept within the concept of Starseeds and the opportunity of extraterrestrial origins. It may be a charming lens via which to discover one's very very very own psychic abilities and spiritual direction.

One of the most important factors of spiritual struggle is retaining a sturdy and notable attitude. This involves that specialize in amazing strength and visualizing a protecting shield round oneself or others. It moreover includes retaining a outstanding attitude and no longer allowing bad mind or feelings to take keep.

Ultimately, religious warfare is ready the usage of one's psychic abilties and religious practices to protect oneself and others from horrible energies and entities. By staying targeted, excessive best, and level-headed, psychics can effectively defend in opposition to non secular assaults and preserve a strong feel of non secular safety.

I encourage you to retain exploring the distinct techniques and practices stated in this ebook, and to by no means prevent reading and growing to your psychic adventure. Remember that psychic abilties may be a powerful tool for personal growth, restoration, and supporting others.

I need that this e-book has supplied you with treasured data and perception into the captivating international of psychic competencies.

Conclusion of contents:

Psychic Abilities: In this section, I added the concept of psychic competencies and cited some of the common ideals and misconceptions about them.

Psychic Energy: This segment explored the concept of psychic power, which consist of what it's far, the way it really works, and the manner it could be tapped into to beautify psychic competencies. I moreover cited the exclusive sorts of psychic energy and the severa capabilities which are associated with them.

Grounding and Raising Vibration: This section provided strategies for grounding into the earth to elevate vibration and beautify psychic skills. I referred to the importance of grounding in shielding oneself from horrible energy and how it could help to enhance psychic capabilities.

Auramagnet Theory: This segment explored the idea of listening to geomagnetic sun storms and how they're capable of have an impact on the body and psychic powers. I brought the Auramagnet Theory, which indicates that the ones solar storms can effect psychic capabilities and offer an possibility for people to beautify their psychic competencies.

Psychic Defense Spells: This phase furnished an extensive evaluation of psychic defense spells, along side what they will be, how they work, and their importance in shielding oneself from terrible strength and psychic attacks. I moreover indexed a number of the superb psychic protection spells and a manner to apply them.

Psychic Love Spells: This phase explored the idea of psychic love spells, at the side of what they will be, how they paintings, and their functionality benefits. I stated some of the fine psychic love spells and a way to use them to attract love and deliver a lift to relationships.

Psychic Success Spells: This phase furnished a pinnacle level view of psychic achievement spells, collectively with what they may be, how they paintings, and their capability blessings. I noted some of the fine psychic fulfillment spells and the way to use them to gain achievement in super areas of life.

Psychic Tools: This phase explored the best-of-a-kind psychic gadget which can be available, such as crystals, tarot gambling playing cards, and sigils. I stated the severa makes use of and benefits of each device, further to the way to use them to decorate psychic abilties.

Trauma-Related Psychic Stress: This segment explored the hyperlink amongst trauma and psychic pressure, which embody how worrying reviews can effect psychic skills. I furnished strategies for dealing with trauma-related psychic strain and methods to beautify healing.

Possession: This segment discussed the symptoms of possession and the results of terrible psychic safety. I explored some of the awesome techniques for defensive oneself from bad energy and psychic assaults, similarly to the manner to deal with ownership if it occurs.

Generational Psychics: This segment explored the concept of generational psychics, collectively with what they will be, how they paintings, and examples of famous generational psychics.

The Bridge among Psychic and the Veil: This phase explored the concept of the veil and the way it pertains to psychic competencies. I referred to strategies for gaining access to the veil and improving psychic skills via the use of meditation and other practices.

Western Zodiac: This section explored each astrological sign and their top notch-recounted psychic tendencies. I mentioned the importance of each signal and their functionality for reinforcing psychic abilities.

Natal Charts: This phase explored the unique homes in a natal chart and a way to apply them for enhancing psychic talents. I stated the importance of each house and how it relates to one in every of a kind regions of existence.

Mayan Astrology: This segment explored the Mayan astrology tool and the way it could be used to beautify psychic abilities. I cited the importance of diverse Mayan symbols and the manner they relate to unique factors of existence.

Chinese Zodiac: This phase explored the Chinese zodiac and the manner it relates to psychic abilties. I cited the importance of each

Tibetan Astrology- This phase explored Tibetan Culture and how it relates to persona inclinations supporting important activities that might guide Clair-talents.

Arabic and Islamic Astrology- additionally called Arabic or Islamic horoscope, is a tool of astrology that originated in the medieval Islamic international and it explored the versions over a long chart.

Native American Astrology- In its hobby- the translation may be shifted amongst tribes and different close by lands.

Egyptian Astrology- Each of those animal totems is related to particular individual inclinations, strengths, weaknesses, and life path traits. For instance, humans born below the Nile totem are stated to be touchy, intuitive, modern, and feature a deep connection to their feelings, whilst those born below the Anubis totem are believed to be clever, analytical, and function strong non secular and psychic skills.

Babylonian Astrology- Babylonian astrology, also referred to as Chaldean astrology, turn out to be one of the earliest types of astrology practiced in ancient Mesopotamia. It modified into advanced round a thousand BCE and grow to be carefully recommended via Sumerian and Akkadian cultures. Babylonian astrology became primarily based on the remark of celestial items, particularly the movements of the planets, and their have an effect on on human affairs.

Chapter 8: Are Mediums And Psychics The Identical Element?

Many human beings use the terms "psychics" and "mediums" and anticipate they propose the same aspect, however the distinction is huge however however so clean to understand.

To me the word "psychic" describes a full-size variety of senses and perceptions which exceed our ordinary physical senses of being attentive to, flavor, sight, contact, and odor.

Psychics receive records approximately human beings and activities from the vibrational electricity of a person, area, or object. A psychic can "take a look at a person's energy" and might apprehend past, present, or destiny occasions in that man or woman's existence.

A medium communicates right now with spirits and connects within the equal manner as a psychic, however rather than reading the strength of the person, they examine the energy of the spirit, they're capable of do that in many strategies, they may pay attention, flavor, see, revel in, and odor additionally called "the Clair's" some mediums can talk with all "the Clair's" and different honestly one or .

So, the wonderful way to give an explanation for the distinction is.

"Psychics understand subjects, Mediums are encouraged/confirmed topics."

What are "the Clair's"?

You may also have heard the terms "clairvoyant" or "clairsentient" however what do they imply? Well permit's make it high-quality and smooth, I've already informed you that some mediums can see, pay interest, flavor, feel and scent, well over time they were given fancy names (that I don't frequently use)

It's very smooth.

The time period Clair comes from French "Clair" that means "clean".

Clairvoyance.

The word Clairvoyance imply smooth-seeing or your inner-imaginative and prescient. A lot of mediums are called clairvoyants, that means they're able to see subjects that other cant, but to me a clairvoyant is a person who can see a verbal exchange in pix or perhaps a presented photo inside the room,

Clairaudience.

The literal translation is apparent-taking note of and may be defined as inner-listening to, this is whilst the connection you are speaking with suggests you through sounds, this will sense discover it impossible to resist's interior your personal mind and naked to the ear. But a few humans also can pay interest it on the "outdoor" inside the room.

Clairsentience.

Clairsentience is likewise referred to as Clear-feeling, I may want to describe it as an inner revel in of some factor that isn't physical, this is frequently emotions or memory triggers, it's that feeling of a 6th feel which you virtually comprehend how a few component feels without touching it.

Clairscent.

Clairsecent is the most not unusual "Clair" and virtually manner clean-heady scent, this is the only that maximum people have expert, You odor some trouble that you apprehend is not within the room or place you're in.

Clairgustance.

Again, allow's keep this easy, it's a unique capacity to revel in taste with out the real presence of meals or drink.

Claircognizance.

Clear-understanding, is that feeling of expertise something without knowing why or how you have got the facts. This is the maximum used Clair for psychic readings. Many people call this Clair "Gut Feeling".

I discover that on the equal time as you start to your journey of development, it is not suitable to get slowed down by prolonged phrases you do not understand. By retaining it clean and decrease decrease returned to fundamentals, you may create a higher know-how of the way you work. Ask your self, "Do I see, pay interest, enjoy, flavor, or heady scent?

Chapter 9: Energy First!

All psychic and spiritual paintings involves strength. It is the maximum easy detail of our existence for the cause that lengthy in advance than the day we landed inside the global plane at beginning and lengthy after we pass lower again to spirit. Empowering your own strength may be very crucial and you may need to recognize and make yourself acquainted along aspect your very own electricity, as well as the energy round you. With the facts and manipulate of power, we are able to be capable of improvement to your course greater without problems, benefit new talents, and apprehend the hidden gives.

What is electricity?

"Energy" is an unseen strain that consists of the visible and unseen worldwide round us. This is maximum generally referred to as everyday power. Despite the dearth of measurable proof for this force, truely every body who has labored with electricity should have had a subjective enjoy.

How you will sense or see this "strength"

•An unseen pressure.

•A warmness or tingling sensation.

•Seeing and feeling solar shades.

•Change of temperature.

•A exchange in popularity.

•Suddenly feeling sick.

•Seeing subjects skip out of the corner of your eye.

•Problems with electric powered gadgets.

Just to name a number of the severa strategies that energy can be confirmed to us.

To artwork with energy, we want to comprehend the essential standards to make it paintings.

The first detail we must do to start operating with power is to turn out to be privy to its life. Remember, "Energy is anywhere." Behind each object and man or woman is an atom, and on the lower back of every atom is electricity. And it can be shown in such lots of approaches.

For example,

the energy of the solar can have a different belongings than the energy of water. The solar has a heat feeling, however notwithstanding the truth that water will experience cool, as they circulate at wonderful speeds.

Exposing your self to positive people will make you stressful while others make you calm, regardless of the truth that you are a distance faraway from them. Again, this is the strength of the individual you experience or being confirmed with the aid of way of manner of the character in the occasion that they are aware about it or no longer.

Energy is independent, is aware about no human criminal tips or ethics. Indeed, it is smart however impartial. And I recollect this is the most vital message to keep in mind whilst we are connecting with strength, our very very own, others, the region spherical us, or possibly the spirit worldwide.

Exercise 1. Sensing Energy.

When beginning on the route of turning into a psychic or a medium, I discover this exercise the most crucial of all, and you could discover that I talk about your private power and the power spherical you in all the carrying activities on this development e book. Before we begin running with our psychic or mediumship energies, we need to recognize our very very personal power and the energy spherical us.

Own energy.

Let's preserve it clean! Look at your self in a reflect and consider how you feel at the identical time as you are glad with love or the feeling of ache in grief? This is the feeling deep interior and now not what you be conscious on your personal expression. Sometimes what we see isn't the actual feeling.

Then ask your self, wherein do you commonly experience it? Find that part of you that feels the emotion, anything emotion that can be. Some human beings feel happy in the coronary heart, and others get that tremendous butterfly feeling within the tummy. And in relation to grief, a few can also experience dizzy, while others sense unwell.

That a part of you is your emotion, and in which you experience your emotions is in that you revel in YOUR OWN strength. Everyone is unique, and there may be no right or incorrect. The more you apprehend your very personal energy, the better you can apprehend the messages you obtain even as we start operating with our psychic/mediumship capabilities.

Sensing Energy inside the Environment.

Let's hold this clean. When we touch something, we interact with it, and we're usually interacting with and touching the surroundings. This way we are commonly sensing electricity. This is why we need to apprehend the surroundings spherical us. I don't recommend the whole international or universe; I actually imply the room or region we are in at that 2nd in time. But endure in thoughts, that is continuously converting due to the truth we are commonly shifting.

Touch is connection.

Look at your toes. Are you barefoot and are your feet touching the floor, or are you wearing socks? You will experience a one-of-a-type sensation for every sort of ground or sock you placed on. You can also moreover get a vibrational sense or, as for me, it might be a enjoy of goosebumps, of anything energy you revel in. It also may be bloodless or warmth, snug, or hard.

For instance,

a rug need to have a surely one in every of a type sensation than grass or a timber floor. So, we're able to mention that the rug has a unique electricity than the grass or the wood floor. (You need to sense along with your complete frame, now not just the textures of the ground.) But for now, don't forget how your selected room or pair of socks make you feel. This snug power may be useful afterward your development.

As you switch out to be higher with sensing the energy of the environment, you could begin to experience the energy while now not having to physical contact the environment. We can walk into the room and get a enjoy of what the strength of the surroundings is like.

For example,

on foot into a quiet vicinity has a exclusive experience, nearly a non violent feeling in contrast to the place of work. The place of job has a extremely good experience than a public coffee keep. Ask your self the manner you experience in the first rate environments, and another time take into account that feeling as it turns into beneficial as you preserve to your path.

We have all walked into an hassle. You can feel the depth within the air, and it's miles very obvious. But are you capable to inform if an difficulty has took place earlier than you even arrived? We can exercising this skills virtually so we also can feel the diffused elements of our environment.

Practice this feel: sense your environment bodily together along with your toes and get a experience of the energy as you stroll into unique environments. We all get that gut feeling; that is the power round you.

But preserve in mind that you are truely staring at and not bringing your very personal feelings into the combination.

Exercise 2. Creating Energy.

To help you understand how electricity works and the way we're capable of interact with it, allow's have a hint amusing and spot if you can shape electricity.

Step One

The first issue and most essential trouble is to lighten up.

Sit without difficulty along side your arms resting for your thighs, palms down.

Inhale very slowly out of your diaphragm, it is below your chest, and exhale slowly.

This might also moreover take some moments, but the extra on top of things of your respiratory you're, the more manipulate you have got of your very very own power.

Step Two

When you are comfortable, deliver each your fingers earlier as if you are protecting a ball with both fingers.

The fingers should slightly face each unique. Focus all your interest on each your fingers at the equal time.

Stay focused and keep all your interest for your fingers, you may start to enjoy a warmness sensation or a tingling sensation on every of your arms.

Step Three

Once you revel in this transformation of sensation, attention your interest in this new sensation (the gap among the hands) on the same time as still sending strength to both hands. By doing this, you are intensifying the modern-day day sensation and moreover you need to feel the energy develop, and the feeling can boom.

Step Four

Now out of your palms, be given as authentic with a beam of moderate, like a laser, emitting from your arms through the space of your fingers. You also can believe a ball of mild amongst your hands. Some people will begin to see the moderate or a change of coloration a few of the palms, so don't fear if you don't. What's essential is feeling the power exchange. As you have got were given have been given commenced to create your non-public energy.

The technique of feeling power may be tough and overwhelming at the start, and it is commonplace to sense discouraged in case you do no longer choose it up right now. However, it's far crucial to remember that everybody's revel in with electricity is unique and there may be no right or wrong way to sense it. Consistency and exercising are key additives in building a stronger connection for your strength and the electricity spherical you. As you continue to paintings in this capability, be affected man or woman with yourself and believe that you can develop your non-public techniques of sensing and deciphering power.

Chapter 10: Am I Psychic?

Psychic abilties and psychic powers permit you to have perceptions past the bodily body. But how do you recognize when you have psychic talents?

Most human beings have idea about this question ultimately in our lives. Maybe within the future you find out that you have very smooth instinct, every other day you could enjoy Deja vu and at yet again you enjoy a colourful dream or maybe clairvoyance.

Some folks are greater psychic than others however we're all born psychics. When it involves developing psychic capabilities, every body enlarge at fantastic speeds, and some can increase extra than others; however all of us own the capacity of being psychic with the proper schooling and techniques.

Psychic capabilities are in reality a 'form of intelligence'; you could look at them in the identical manner you discover ways to energy or play a musical tool. You genuinely discover ways to positioned the things in the appropriate order and the manner to recognize your very personal feelings.

One of the maximum not unusual questions in psychic development is how are you going to tell if what you got, or sense is certainly psychic or truly natural creativeness?

A psychic affect may be very one-of-a-kind from the everyday feeling given from our very own imagination. At first the emotions are normally random and spontaneous that regularly come without caution however with practice can emerge as centered.

They show themselves in such pretty some methods together with a gut feeling, visions, premonitions or maybe understanding a few problem about a person's beyond with out being informed, you can even feel how the person is feeling, you could had been in an amazing mood till they walked inside the room, otherwise you get a chilly shiver, and that they pop into your thoughts.

We don't must be sat in a darkish candlelit room to get preserve of messages, or perhaps be with the individual the message is for, and this is the motive it's difficult to inform the difference among us being psychic or certainly our imagination. But the greater you exercise, the higher you will recognize the "psychic feeling", so you recognize on the same time as you are receiving messages or really overthinking.

We are all psychic in first-rate strategies, it's far developing the expertise of the way we paintings (accumulate information) that is the present, the prevailing is not being a psychic.

So, the answer on your query is....

"Yes, we are all psychic, however some are extra effective than others."

How will the psychic impressions be confirmed to me?

These impressions can take vicinity in masses of methods, collectively with via goals, visions, or unexpected insights. Sometimes they come , flooding the mind with a wealth of information, while extraordinary instances they arrive in dribs and drabs, revealing themselves one impact at a time. No rely how they come, the ones impressions are powerful device that may assist us to advantage belief into the world spherical us and to tap into our private ranges of instinct.

Forms of impressions:

Feelings of randomness or spontaneous mind.

Interruption of your everyday teach of concept.

Persistent nagging feeling.

Strong feelings with memories behind it.

Reoccurring visions.

Seeing the identical symbols time and again again which includes 1111 or 1212.

Seeing and feeling colorations.

Change of temperature.

Just to call some!

Remember, the existing is understanding how you figure, and also you couldn't enjoy any of the above or you could have them each single day. There isn't any right or incorrect close to walking at the aspect of your personal psychic ability.

What shape of facts may be confirmed to me?

This is a very tough query to answer but here is a list of the maximum commonplace.

The past and gift.

Family

Possible future plans/direction

Life records

Recent life changes

Hobbies/ hobbies

Life commands

Former or new relationships

This list is ever lasting.

We additionally may be verified matters round the area from wars to disasters,

Exercise three. The Psychic Test.

This smooth check is a notable region to start your psychic journey , however at this degree, I'm not going to offer an motive behind a few element .So permit's get commenced.

What you may need.

A buddy / family member or perhaps a stranger. (We call them the sitter)

A black pen

Paper

An envelope

You!

Step One

Ask your pal, family member, or stranger "the sitter" to attract a clean, childlike face of the manner they're feeling or felt that day. Ask them to make it easy: dots for eyes, one dot for the nose, and a line for the mouth.

Then, with out you looking on the drawing, ask them to vicinity it face down in the envelope on the table in the front of you.

Step Two

It's time to loosen up.

Sit with out a problem collectively together with your fingers resting in your thighs, palms down.

Inhale very slowly from your diaphragm, it is under your chest, and exhale slowly.

This can also take some moments, however the more on pinnacle of factors of your respiration you're, the more manipulate you've got got over your personal strength.

Step Three

Get to understand yourself and the surroundings round you. How do you feel?

What's the strength like? Is the area you are in making you feel cushty?

Once you revel in you recognize your very non-public feelings and the region spherical you, it's now time to begin the check.

Step Four

Focus all of your energy on the envelope with out touching it. In your thoughts, use the power to touch the cardboard. Some human beings will see a slight, and others will see not anything however will revel in the electricity. Make a examine in case you see or experience something.

Ask the strength to draw the face in your thoughts or ask it to make you sense the emotion of the face at the paper. Do you notice a grin or revel in unhappy? At this stage, don't fear in case you don't see or experience some thing, but make a phrase in case you do.

Now it's your turn to draw a face with out pronouncing a few element to the sitter, then area it face down next to the envelope.

Step Five

Place your left hand at the envelope and your right hand on your drawing.

Inhale very slowly out of your diaphragm and exhale slowly.

Ask yourself do they sense the identical or is there a change of anergy?

Step six

It's time to look how you likely did, did you manipulate to draw the identical image, and did you enjoy the emotion? Open the envelope and feature a glance.

What did I simply do?

In this exercising, we are walking out how you figure as a psychic. Some people are empathic, because of this that they enjoy electricity. This may be a pressure or an emotion, and others see electricity. This can be colored lights or snap shots inside the thoughts or inside the environment spherical us. Many people ought to name this a gift, however to me, knowledge how we psychically art work is "the gift."

Ask your self, did I see a few aspect, or did I feel it? If you did not revel in a few element or see a few issue, do the experiment over again, however this time, at the same time as you get to step four, ask the power to reveal you thru feelings, and make a be privy to the manner you felt. Did you experience heat or bloodless, and did you revel in happy or unhappy?

If you did now not revel in a few component, start all all over again, and at step four, ask the power to show you. Did you see shades inside the room or a face to your thoughts? Are the colors warm or cool colorations, and what do the colors make you sense? Or did you notice a smiley face or a tear in a watch fixed?

Now you've got were given the basics, you may do this exercising the usage of different drawings. Ask the sitter to draw a shape or location a playing card within the envelope. This workout is a great way of information electricity, and the extra you exercising, the better you will become.

Exercise 4. Psychic Colours.

Any decorator or fashion dressmaker will will let you realize that how critical shade is in our lives…The hues round us can trade our moods, make us more or heaps lots less lively, productive, amorous, or possibly glamorous.

So, it shouldn't be a wonder that we use colorings whilst we art work with psychic power. In the subsequent exercise, we will start to create our very very very own psychic shade chart.

What you need.

Paper

Red pen/pencil

Orange pen/pencil

Yellow pen/pencil

Green pen/ pencil

Blue pen/pencil

Purple pen/pencil

Pink pen/pencil

Black pen/pencil

You!

Step One

Using the purple pen/pencil, draw a small square at the left aspect of the paper and positioned the pen down.

Step Two

It's time to loosen up.

Sit quite simply collectively with your arms resting in your thighs, arms down. Inhale very slowly out of your diaphragm, that is beneath your chest, and exhale slowly.

This might also moreover additionally take some moments, however the more on pinnacle of things of your respiration you are, the extra manipulate you have got over your non-public power.

Step Three

Focus all of your power on the "Red Square" and ask yourself how that Colour makes you revel in.

Step Four

Write the primary 3 terms/emotions that come to mind.

Step Five

Repeat all of the steps with the alternative coloured pens.

Congratulations

You have truly created your personal simple emotion coloration chart. This chart may be a few detail that can be used as a reference while operating collectively together with your psychic strength, and once more, the extra you use it, the less difficult it becomes.

When you revel in extra snug, you may increase for your colour chart through which include extra shades or maybe solar sun shades however hold in mind to hold it clean.

Here is a color chart for manual capabilities satisfactory and I propose taking time to create your private.

Here is an instance of an stepped forward colour chart.

RED.

BRIGHT. Passionate, Strong, Courageous, Luck, Happiness, Richness, Excitement, Bold, Extrovert, Alive, Activation.

DARK. Fierce, Oppressive, Vindictive, Aggressive, Rage, Danger, Stop, Frustration

ORANGE.

BRIGHT. Warm Optimism, Energy, Protection, Lightness, Joy, Pleasure, Relaxed, Calm.

DARK. Ambition, Pride, Sickly, Selfishness

YELLOW.

BRIGHT. Sun, Awake, Uplifted, Learning, Balance, Inspirational, Communication

DARK. Guidance, Insecure, Loss, Irritable

GREEN.

BRIGHT. Balance, Nature, Harmony, Earth, Versatile, Clear, Judgement,

DARK- Envy, Jealousy, Betrayal, Indecision, Illness

BLUE

BRIGHT – Peace, Healing, Cool, Sympathy, Understanding, Nursing, Relaxing, Calmness, Quiet, Settled

DARK- Deep philosopher, Withdrawn, Shy, Worry, Depression

PURPLE

BRIGHT- Loyal, Intuitive, Spiritual, Solitude, Mediation, Concentration

DARK- Introvert, Unbalanced, Uneasy

PINK

BRIGHT- Love, Family, Empathy, Open minded

DARK- Deep harm, Emotion, Power

Exercise five. It's a signal.

There are signs and symptoms and signs and symptoms and logos for nearly everything in existence, together with doves for peace, horseshoes for proper fortune, flags for international places, pink hearts for romance, animals for well-known individual signs, or even feathers for spirit. In regular existence, we use symptoms and symbols to talk with each specific with out the spoken phrase. Most symbols additionally evoke an emotion. Let's take the commonplace sign for sure. With your hand-held tight in a fist, you beautify your thumb up so it elements to the sky. This signal can often make you experience delight or happiness, however flip it on its head, and also you revel in upset or uneasy.

From delivery, we are demonstrated symptoms and logos that have extra meanings than simply an movement or maybe a photograph. I name this the photograph dictionary, and every day of our lives, we upload to this magic e-book in our very personal thoughts.

The trouble is we've got become so used to the usage of them that we forget about approximately what they mean. So, we want to take time to remind ourselves earlier than we're able to use them in our psychic art work. This subsequent workout is to make you consider what the power is attempting to reveal you... are you seeing a horseshoe or feeling fortunate?

It's your photograph dictionary and may be very important to go together with your very very own feelings.

What you need.

•Paper

•pen/pencil

Step One

On the left-hand side of the paper, write or draw the subsequent listing.

A Cat.

A horseshoe.

A gold ring.

A white bird.

A tree.

A clock.

A rainbow.

Step Two

Next to the image/sign, write what it approach to you,

For example,

Horseshoe – Luck

Step Three

Next to the outline, write the number one 3 terms or emotions that come to mind.

Horseshoe - Luck - Happy/Relaxed/Feet.

Congratulations

You have virtually commenced to create your very own Picture dictionary. This dictionary will certainly evolve as you do, and each time you see a few problem make a highbrow word of it or write it down.

When I say make a be conscious

I need you to look and revel in the energy of the photograph,

Ask yourself "What come to be it I noticed?" "What did it suggest?" And "how did it make me revel in?"

One sign/symbol can recommend greater than surely one component and will have a selected which means to me than it's going to to you.

The electricity of symbols is charming. They have the capability to rouse feelings, reminiscences, and meanings that adjust from man or woman to character. What can also additionally look like a smooth photo to at the least one, can hold a big cost to some other. In my case, the symbol of a crimson bus brought about feelings of adventure and happiness, as I reminisced my travels in London.

However, to someone else, the same picture also can want to hold a one-of-a-type significance. For instance, someone who grew up taking the bus to school every day can also companion the purple bus with memories of youth and recurring. Or someone who's a die-tough Harry Potter fan can also moreover furthermore see the equal photograph and don't forget the well-known scene wherein Harry, Ron, and Hermione take the Knight Bus to interrupt out from danger.

That's one of the maximum first-rate subjects about symbols. They can hold multiple meanings and can be interpreted in wonderful processes. They have a established language that may be felt and understood with the beneficial useful resource of many, but even though maintain individual importance. It's awesome how a easy photograph can be part of us to memories, people, and opinions that mean a lot to us.

It's your that means that's important.

Exercise 6. Putting it together.

In the ultimate 3 sporting events, we looked at how we artwork as a psychic. In Exercise three, The Psychic Test, we asked ourselves, "Did we see or experience power?" Then, in Exercise four, you need to have commenced out to paintings with sunglasses and the manner they made you sense, and what that shade supposed to you. In Exercise five, you started out making your very very non-public photo dictionary. Now, it's time to put all of them together.

What you will need.

A p.C. Of playing gambling playing playing cards

A black pen/pencil

Paper

Step One

Yet again, it's time to loosen up.

Sit efficaciously together along with your arms resting on your thighs, hands down.

Inhale very slowly out of your diaphragm, this is below your chest, and exhale slowly.

This may also take a few moments, but the greater on pinnacle of things of your respiratory you're, the extra manage you have got got got of your very very own power.

Step Two

Get to recognize your self and the surroundings round you. How do you experience? What's the energy like? Is the area you are in making you experience comfortable? Once you revel in you apprehend your personal emotions and the location round you, it's now time to begin the check.

Step Three

Shuffle the % of playing cards and consciousness all of your electricity on the playing cards. In your mind, use the electricity to touch the playing playing playing cards. Some people will see a mild, and others will see nothing however will enjoy the strength.

Step Four

As you attention your power on the entire deck of playing gambling playing cards, pick a single card out of the deck and region it face down in the the front of you. Do now not check it. Place the relaxation of the deck a ways from you. It is important that they're no longer within the front of you or next to the single card. The complete deck now holds your strength, and we don't need it to have an effect to your psychic quit end result.

Step Five.

At this degree, it is crucial to Ask Questions. This will assist you stay targeted and in control of the workout.

Ask the cardboard, "What coloration are you? (Red? Black?)" Write the coloration down.

Tips: Remind your self what the two colorings endorse to you. Look again at your colour chart.

Ask the cardboard, "What form are you? (Heart? Diamond? Spade? Club?)" Write the form down.

Tip: Look again at your image dictionary. Have you seen the shape or are you inquisitive about some component spherical you?

Ask the cardboard, "What are you? (1-10? Jack? King? Queen? Ace? — 1 and ace are the equal card)" Write it down.

Tip: look at your palms what number of hands do you want to hold up? Or are you seeing/feeling a photograph — make a be privy to what you notice as that is you which includes to your very personal image dictionary.

Step Six

How did you do?

Don't circulate a few one of a kind playing playing cards, in reality the unmarried card this is facedown. Turn it over and let's have a look at how you probably did. Did you get the colour proper? Did you apprehend if it modified proper right into a coronary coronary heart, diamond, spade, or club? And did you get the extensive variety or image accurate?

Congratulations

If you controlled to get all three correct, however if you didn't, don't worry. Let's see if the surroundings has impacted your analyzing.

At the start, I requested you to region the entire deck of cards to as a minimum one aspect, turn over the pinnacle card of the p.C., and examine your consequences. Again, what number of out of three did you get? Now do the same with the lowest card. This will show you in case you need more interest and is a brilliant "decrease again to fundamentals" exercise.

I suggest doing this exercising as often as you may. You will find out it's first-rate to easy the thoughts and truly interesting. And at the identical time as you sense comfortable, you are extra at one collectively collectively with your very personal energy.

Chapter 11: Am I A Medium?

When most people think about mediums, they recollect an old female in an extended flowing skirt who is a piece normal, and all of the children in the location dare each super to knock on the door earlier than running away. Well, I hate to burst that bubble, however I'm no longer an antique woman, and youngsters are not fearful of me. I'm only a regular individual, much like anyone else.

Being a medium approach having the capability to hook up with the spirit worldwide. Most humans have the misconception that mediums speak to "the lifeless," however the fact is, most mediums can't pay attention spirits.

There are many techniques to talk with spirits. Some human beings name the techniques we communicate "the Clairs," but I want to preserve it smooth. Some mediums pay interest, see, revel in, scent, and taste at the same time as speaking with spirits. Some mediums, like me, have the ability to do all, however maximum mediums can best do one or a number of "the Clairs."

There also are some brilliant sorts of medium, the intellectual medium and the physical medium.

A intellectual medium is the most not unusual medium, someone who's able to speak with spirit whilst they'll be aware via seeing, listening to, feeling, smelling, or tasting.

Physical Mediumship is not as common nowadays as it have grow to be in Victorian instances and the early 20th century. The varieties of Physical phenomena typically encountered are Transfiguration, Ectoplasm, Voice Trumpets, Materialization, and Apports.

I remember that each toddler is born a medium, but we're conditioned through life and overlook what we were born with. We are knowledgeable it's ordinary, uncommon, or maybe horrifying. But with the right training and assist, we can open up what we can also have closed off or begin noticing subjects we once omitted.

So, what makes you believe you studied you could a medium?

You get highbrow photographs.

One example of this is whilst a person is speakme to you approximately a deceased family member, and you get a mental flash of what that character appeared like while not having them defined to you. Or, for no purpose, you observe a face to your thoughts, just like a photograph.

You can scent fragrances which aren't sincerely gift.

Have you ever walked into a room and glued a whiff of perfume or probable the nasty scent of a cigarette or cigar, and nobody else seems to word it?

You enjoy much like the air is suddenly whole of electricity that makes you sense superb.

This is one of those signs and symptoms and signs and symptoms that can sincerely make you question your sanity earlier than you learn how to recognize what is going on.

Seeing topics go together with the go with the flow out of the corner of your eye.

Many human beings have professional seeing a few issue skip out of the corner of their eye, excellent to turn and find out that now not some element is there. For mediums, this may be a greater ordinary phenomenon than for the commonplace man or woman.

Walking into a few places reasons you to get a headache.

You can also sense a heaviness or exclusive sensations, or even feelings. Sometimes you would likely get a headache. This may be disconcerting, even while you are acquainted along with your present, but especially in the starting.

Are you frightened of the darkish?

Many mediums have had a fear of the darkish at one issue or another in their lives. Okay, many children have a worry of the darkish.

 television's, radios or maybe lighting move on and stale on their private.

This can stand up at any time of the day, and lots of mediums may be involved approximately this physical interplay.

 Is it cold in right here?

You also can get a rush of cold or warmness air passing with the resource of way of you.

 You experience someone, or a few issue touch you.

You understand that you are home on my own, and suddenly, some aspect strokes your hair or nips your bottom. You turn around to discover no individual status within the lower back of you.

 Did you name me?

You pay interest your call being known as in random locations. You may be walking down the road of a city you have got never been to in advance than, and a person calls your call. Or you could be inside the tub, and also you concentrate your call being referred to as out, so that you call lower again first-rate to be knowledgeable no one shouted your name.

The most not unusual questions in mediumship.

How are you able to tell if what you bought, or revel in is really from Spirit or simply pure creativeness?

A mediumistic impact can experience similar to our personal imagination and can be tough to interpret, however fear no longer, there are carrying activities you could do to help you and the spirit global speak in a manner you every apprehend. At first, the feelings are generally random and spontaneous, and often come without caution, but with exercise, they could end up focused.

What records will the spirit worldwide deliver me?

Again that may be a definitely tough query to reply but here is a list of the maximum not unusual

The beyond and gift.

Family.

Possible future plans/course.

Life statistics.

Recent lifestyles adjustments.

Hobbies/ pursuits.

Life commands.

Former or new relationships.

How someone died.

What they seemed like.

The pain they felt.

But most of all love.

The spirit worldwide is an elusive realm in which communication is frequently random and unpredictable. While many people want to get preserve of specific messages from their cherished ones who have handed away, it is critical to understand that the spirit worldwide operates otherwise from the physical worldwide. This technique that the information that spirits carry to us won't commonly align with our expectancies or dreams. We need to don't forget that spirits have restrained electricity and time to talk with us, so they will not usually cope with the topics that we need to talk about.

To establish a reference to the spirit international, it is crucial to invite questions and engage in conversation. By asking spirits questions, we are capable of manual the verbal exchange closer to the subjects that depend to us at the same time as moreover respecting the regulations of their energy. This method permits us to set up a greater big reference to the spirit global, and it increases the possibility of receiving applicable messages from our loved ones. Overall, growing a deeper information of the spirit global calls for staying power, open-mindedness, and a willingness to encompass unexpected communique.

Setting Intention.

Before we start operating with the spirit international, we must set the purpose, which means that we've got to inform them and ourselves that we are geared up to artwork. This is the right time for them to show us they're there, and you're on pinnacle of factors of the relationship.

This additionally permits us manipulate the relationship and could prevent random thoughts and "leaping" connections.

I assume it is very vital to first-class paintings with spirits while you're prepared or what some may additionally name "open." And certain, it sincerely is proper, we must no longer be open all the time. You are in control of your verbal exchange with the spirit international, now not the opportunity way round. Many human beings do no longer recognize if or even as they're connecting. By placing this purpose, you recognize what to be looking for. At the equal time, you're telling the spirit worldwide when they need to soar forward.

How can we set purpose?

Intention is the essential first step closer to large communication. It includes a conscious choice to acquire out and be a part of. By starting ourselves up, what I call selecting up the cellphone and taking it off the answering cell phone, we signal our willingness to interact and recognize, and to create region for mutual exchange. Whether it's far through a proper greeting or a 2d of silent pondered picture, expressing our purpose to mixture devices the tone for a effective verbal exchange. Some call this an opening message or a prayer, to me it is simple - it's far only some terms of apprehend announcing, "allow's communicate".

Some human beings will send a idea out to their very personal spirit courses, protectors or possibly God, but I surely enjoy that this "Let's speak" should be open to the divine and ever-loving spirit.

Here is a small message of goal.

Divine and ever-loving spirits,

Could the most effective and the brightest come beforehand to show us that we aren't on my own and to remind us that we might not be capable of see you every day, however you live on round us? I do this with recognize and count on recognize in pass again. This is the right time to talk with me, and I will can help you apprehend once I have completed. This message is to remind you that I am on pinnacle of things of our connection. I thank you earlier with love and mild.

Amen.

I recognise the message sounds a touch strongly worded, however it's you empowering yourself, then reminding the spirit international who's in rate. It's normally completed with admire, but if we failed to set the purpose, the spirit global might anticipate we preferred to talk with them while we have to now not or whilst we don't have anybody to pass the message directly to.

You can make your very own message of intention however take into account to maintain it easy and continually with understand to the spirit global, but maximum of all to your self.

Closing off to the spirit international

The idea of remaining off is once more an goal of ending verbal exchange with the spirit international spherical us. If we failed to near off or vicinity the phone on silent/answer mobile smartphone, we'd be open to verbal exchange 24 hours a day, 7 days consistent with week, three hundred and sixty five days a year, and the spirit global might be trying to chat at each possibility.

The maximum essential reasons for final conversation are:

You are on top of things, Its recognize for your self, Its recognize for special human beings around you,

But most of all its, so you recognize even as you are receiving a message and it's now not definitely your non-public random mind,

How to close a message/ save you verbal exchange until you're ready to start walking all over again.

Divine and ever-loving spirits,

Thank you for displaying me which you useful resource my spiritual art work and which you accept as true with in me, but now I send all the moderate and love once more to you, as I pass back to my ordinary lifestyles. I remind you that this is my time and my life, so with apprehend, please step decrease back till I ship the message of affection and ask for communication. Once another time, I thanks in your conversation, with love and mild.

Amen.

THIS IS THE MOST IMPORTANT MESSAGE YOU WILL EVER SEND TO SPIRIT!

If you discover that spirit is round you after you have got were given stated this message, don't worry. Don't be amazed if it emerge as you that invited them in without noticing. Did you notice some thing and say, "what's that," or scent a few issue and say, "who's there"?

Remember, smooth phrases can open verbal exchange.

www.ingramcontent.com/pod-product-compliance
Lightning Source LLC
Chambersburg PA
CBHW071446080526
44587CB00014B/2008